Iboogane (+ run into Lundy)

Essay on K___
Scientific bt___
poetic + personal

Title of book

Dopamine

Sleep interrupted + poor
woke a bit shaky
Tremor — mostly reduced but bad
Walk — ∪
Co-ord — ∪
H — ∪

AS — reduced but present

S — ∪
B — OK

✗ aft/eve best time

Felt tired or overexercised?
Late pill ? too much tea

dyskinesia
dystonia

hypomimia

hypophonia

hyposmia
dystonia .
orthostasis
sialorrhea

Praise for

In This Faulty Machine

"*In This Faulty Machine* is a wonder, a memoir of illness that becomes an affirmation of life and vitality. As Parkinson's seeks to narrow, Kathy Page pushes back, resolved to fully inhabit whatever experience life offers. I read this book in awe and some of it in tears. Intelligent, thoughtful, and candid, *In This Faulty Machine* is destined to be a classic."
—**Joan Thomas, award-winning author of** *Wild Hope* **and** *Five Wives*

"Kathy Page offers an unflinching, beautifully detailed account of life with Parkinson's disease. With raw honesty and a unique perspective, she breathes meaning into the often soulless medical language surrounding the disease. Page explores the profound ways Parkinson's reshapes identity—the grief of what's lost, the slivers of humour that remain, and the quiet resilience that carries her forward. This is not a story

of surrender, but of survival and rediscovery. *In This Faulty Machine* is a moving reminder that while Parkinson's may change you, it does not define you— and that even in the face of loss, we are never without hope or purpose."
—**Bailey Martin, Executive Director, Parkinson Wellness Projects**

"A masterpiece of observation. Animated by Kathy Page's curious and brilliant mind, this chronicle explores the darkest layers of Parkinson's, shining a powerful light into illness. Yet like all truly great books, it makes us feel better about the strange, fragile humans that we are. Honest, tender, joyful, moving, *In This Faulty Machine* is infused with a rare kind of insight that is genuinely healing."
—**Shaena Lambert, award-winning author of *Petra* and *Oh, My Darling***

"Thrust by illness into being the main character in her own medical drama, Kathy Page reflects on her life as a writer and her very existence as a human being. The self-described 'former novelist' pieces together more than enough of her old creative self to turn a sow's ear—the disease that overturned her life—into this silk purse of a memoir."
—**Elizabeth Hay, award-winning and bestselling author of *All Things Consoled* and *Snow Road Station***

"Long one of our best fiction writers, Kathy Page has now written a startling memoir, turning her lively wit and unflinching insight on a cruel twist of fate. . . . Though deeply personal, what she undergoes is universal, for hers is the struggle of everyone for life and love against the end, suddenly sped up. Bold, frank, free from self-pity, this beautifully written book is one of the wisest and most moving I have read."

—Ronald Wright, award-winning author of *A Short History of Progress* and *A Scientific Romance*

"This wondrous memoir is less about coping with disease than a testament to living well and staying open to, and curious about, the complex, unreliable machine that is the body. One of our finest novelists, Page presents her experience of illness with the same wit and generosity of spirit that she brings to her fiction. Her diagnosis, though unenviable, nonetheless brings her, and us, a compensatory richness of love and insight. *In This Faulty Machine* is one of those rare books that compels you to rethink your life."

—Caroline Adderson, award-winning author of *A Way to Be Happy* and *A Russian Sister*

"Wonder and gratitude—how else to feel about the warm intelligence and poise with which Kathy Page tells her story? 'I'm no stoic,' she says, 'but you can't be howling all the time.' And so she marshals her abundant gifts as a novelist—wit, curiosity and compassion, married to an exquisite command of her prose—and invites us into this profound exploration of vulnerability and possibility. A true marvel of a book."

—**John Gould, author of** *The End of Me* **and** *Kilter*

In This Faulty Machine

Also by Kathy Page

~

In This Faulty Machine

A Memoir
of Loss and
Transformation

Kathy Page

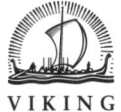

VIKING

VIKING

an imprint of Penguin Canada, a division of Penguin Random House Canada Limited

Canada • USA • UK • Ireland • Australia • New Zealand • India • South Africa • China

First published 2025

Viking, an imprint of Penguin Canada
A division of Penguin Random House Canada
320 Front Street West, Suite 1400
Toronto, Ontario, M5V 3B6, Canada
penguinrandomhouse.ca

The authorized representative in the EU for product safety and compliance is Penguin Random House Ireland, Morrison Chambers, 32 Nassau Street, Dublin D02 YH68, Ireland, https://eu-contact.penguin.ie

Excerpt from Oliver Sacks, *Awakenings* permission "Awakening" from AWAKENINGS by Oliver Sacks, © 1973, Oliver Sacks, used by permission of The Wylie Agency (UK) Limited, and © 1973, 1976, 1982, 1983, 1987, 1990, Oliver Sacks, used by permission of Vintage Books, an imprint of the Knopf Doubleday Publishing Group, a division of Penguin Random House LLC. All rights reserved.

Portions of some chapters have been previously published: "Passport" as "That Other Place" in *The New Quarterly* 160; reprinted in *Best Canadian Essays 2023* ed. Mireille Silcoff, Biblioasis; and "The Exquisite Cyclops" in *Geist* 127

LIBRARY AND ARCHIVES CANADA CATALOGUING IN PUBLICATION

Title: In this faulty machine : a memoir of loss and transformation / Kathy Page.
Names: Page, Kathy, 1958- author
Identifiers: Canadiana (print) 20250158779 | Canadiana (ebook) 20250158795 | ISBN 9781037800887 (hardcover) | ISBN 9781037800894 (EPUB)
Subjects: LCSH: Page, Kathy, 1958—Health. | LCSH: Parkinson's disease—Patients—Canada—Biography. | CSH: Authors, Canadian (English)—21st century—Biography. | LCGFT: Autobiographies.
Classification: LCC RC382 .P34 2025 | DDC 362.1968/330092—dc23

Book design by Andrew Roberts
Typeset by Terra Page
Cover design by Andrew Roberts
Cover images: (red tulip) © kolesnikovserg, (dried tulip) © krstrbrt, both Adobe Stock

Printed in Canada

10 9 8 7 6 5 4 3 2 1

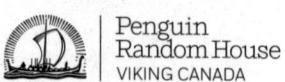

Penguin
Random House
VIKING CANADA

For my sister Jan

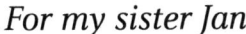

Contents

~

1

~

Passport

In the wake of my horrible diagnosis, as I struggled to make sense of what was happening to me and what lay ahead, the opening of an essay by Susan Sontag, read decades ago, tugged at my memory. I remembered her assertion that being seriously ill was a kind of exile or deportation to another place, the kingdom of the sick. A separation. Other writers before and since have explored, expanded on, and argued with the idea of the kingdom or country of the sick, but there was something, some detail of the way she expressed it that I wanted to recall.

I tracked down *Illness as Metaphor* and found what I was looking for on the first page: the passport. "Although we prefer to use only the good passport, sooner or later each of us is obliged, at least for a spell, to identify ourselves as citizens of that other place." In the light of experience, I could see and feel that not-good, sick person passport as if it had been real. It brought Sontag's cool, almost legalistic words to life, and me to tears.

Cheaply made, its charcoal-grey cover displaying only a biometric chip, the new passport that I imagined was nothing like the two classy and similarly heraldic passports I already possessed: the gold and dark-blue Canadian, and the maroon and gold of the United Kingdom of Great Britain and Northern Ireland, which still for the duration of the post-Brexit transition year allowed me to travel freely anywhere in the European Union.

The grey passport did not confer freedom. Purely restrictive, it contained no space for visas; instead, a few pages of regulations written in tiny hieroglyphic type found on the labels of medications, illegible even when you have your glasses on. A long list of forbidden activities was stapled to the back cover. The stamp, *Indefinite*, made it clear that I was to remain in the kingdom of the sick unless judged by persons and processes unknown to be well again.

I could tell the officer behind the Plexiglas that this must be a mistake. How I have a family who needs me, how I'd never asked for this document, did not fill in any application form, and do not want it. I could weep and beg but she would merely instruct me to look at the scanner.

"Good. Move on." The crowd I was now part of pushed toward distant exit signs. Every kind of language and diversity was there. Elderly, young, even children. Bandages, crutches, wheelchairs. Some looked sick, others not. A small boy with a shaved head slipped his cold, damp hand into mine. Ahead, a row of revolving doors. Pressed into a compartment with too many others, I tried to protect the boy—only to stumble out, alone, into a car park. I was back at the hospital. Almost home! No. That was only the first impression, a cruel twist. Beneath the familiar surfaces, everything had changed.

Kingdom is perhaps too grand and old-fashioned a word for this "other place" in which the sick must live. This simulacrum pretending to be my life is more akin to a modern state, highly bureaucratic, whether totalitarian or merely dysfunctional.

Even the mental kind of travel is forbidden. I'm compelled now to devote almost all of my attention to observing the nature, frequency, intensity, and duration of symptoms: *Unable to do buttons/put lid on jar/ dress in leggings. Hands v. weak. Things with two hands more difficult. Tremors worse. Juddering in arms. Walk: 55 minutes* . . . I've filled several notebooks with scrawled records of this kind, some so faintly written as to be nearly illegible. Such focus is necessary, yet also terribly destructive in the way it monopolizes the mind: the huge, rich, complex world beyond one's body and immediate environment fades at times into a vaguely realized backdrop, a view of something now beyond reach.

As for who and where was I before I had to take up this additional, entirely involuntary citizenship, some things have not changed: I was and always will be the mother of our two children, who were at the time symptoms first showed themselves in their early twenties and beginning to live independent lives. I was and hope to remain happily married to their father, Richard, a man I've loved for a quarter of a century. We lived then as we do now on a rocky, forested, ferry-dependent island with a population of around twelve thousand. We had built a ridge-top house surrounded by a productive kitchen garden and ten acres of trees only a few kilometres away from the main village, a busy, artsy community hub. It's a home we will now leave sooner than intended.

Before the new passport, I could work hard both professionally and domestically. I was halfway through writing my ninth novel. Though neither rich nor famous, I was doing work that mattered to me and to my readers. I travelled regularly to present my books in North America and Europe, and for the past twenty years, I had taught writing part-time at a university on Vancouver Island: fulfilling work which had helped me, a relative newcomer to Canada, become part of the local and wider creative communities.

At the beginning of a new semester, I often spoke to my students about how fortunate I thought we all were to be able to spend even a few hours each week *imagining*. Imagining the daily life of someone they had glimpsed on the bus one morning, or what a character they had already brought to life might do if faced with an impossible-seeming choice (itself to be imagined). How a world or society looked and functioned in granular detail. Likewise, learning an ancient craft: how to make compelling sentences, how to listen to the sounds of words, how to use imagery, all in the cause of constructing stories that might blossom in another person's mind. How lucky we were to have, in an era of spreadsheets and profits before people or planet, time set aside to practise and enjoy the particular and very intense form of human communication and connection that creating and sharing stories offers us.

I did not mention to the students that teaching had brought me good fortune in another way too. Back in 1994 when we both still lived in England, I met my future husband at a community education class I had been hired to teach once a week in an overheated portable classroom on the grounds of a high school in Surbiton, an outer suburb of London.

On the first evening, he was both the last student to arrive and exactly on time. I checked him off the register as he slipped into the remaining plastic chair. To say that I immediately noticed him—tall, slim, his gaze both intense and open as he took in the room and the people in it, how the light sweater he wore fit him perfectly—would be an understatement. I had to make myself look away, and for a minute or two, my voice seemed to belong to someone else.

Relationships between students and teachers are, for good reasons, discouraged, and were so even back in 1994. However, I'm very glad we met. I think we might have waited until after the end of that term before acknowledging the attraction between us, had it not happened, in week seven, that my car was stolen. This forced me to take the train, which made me late for class, and at the end of the evening my husband-to-be drove me to a station halfway to my home, saying it was on his way.

The following week, he offered to drive me all the way home. Still, when he parked outside my flat, I didn't ask him in, though I did kiss him, hurriedly, on the cheek. He offered his phone number. I opened my address book to write it down, and we both saw that it was already there, copied from the register for future use. The way we laughed at this seemed like a good sign.

It all happened quickly after that: sex, food, love, theatre, art galleries, visits to families, travel to Wales, Ireland, Spain, Portugal, France, Morocco. We were both in our mid-thirties. The power balance did not seem to tip consistently in either direction. We had a frank conversation about children. Given our ages, especially mine (thirty-six), we couldn't be sure it would be possible.

We committed to sharing as equally or as fairly as possible the intimate domestic part of life. When our two children came along, we kept to this for both child care and housework, and it is how we've lived, until now. It's an arrangement not everyone would be comfortable with, and one which conventional workplaces and a gendered wage gap make difficult to choose, but we both wanted the same thing, and our luck was such that once we began living together, we had some flexibility. When we met, Richard had recently returned from a year-long adventure with three friends. They had driven a double-decker London bus around the world as a fundraiser for sustainable development charities. In pre-Google days, researching, planning, and organizing this by letter and telephone was a huge, slow, and complex task, which had itself taken two years of Richard's free time. While this circumnavigation earned the crew a place in the Guinness World Records, it had lost Richard his fiancée. A rough patch followed. Now in a supposedly stop-gap job as manager of two designer goods stores owned by a friend, he wanted to start over, to find something that used his mind and imagination. Meanwhile, he could at least control his own hours.

When the children were small, we fixed up a home in scraps of sleep-fogged so-called spare time between paid work and child care. New technologies meant that opportunities for flexible hours teaching from home were beginning to come my way. And I wrote, some days, only for twenty minutes, but even that felt good. The publishing industry was entering a time of huge upheaval and became increasingly focussed on bestsellers. I'd been despondent about the prospects for the kind of writing I wanted to do in this new reality. But as our relationship developed, desire and confidence returned. Having Richard and the children exposed parts of me I had not known existed. It enriched my writing, and on a mundane plane, babies taught me how to make good use of limited time. I rewrote my stalled sixth novel, *The Story of My Face*, with my daughter napping beside my desk.

We were lucky to have found each other, to have conceived so easily. Both children were healthy. Our daughter had arrived after a lengthy labour with the cord looped around her neck. Three years later, our son, not to be outdone, sported five loops around his neck and emerged swiftly by emergency C-section. He suffered no ill effects. But it could have been otherwise. We knew he would be our last and that it was time to settle into the shape of things to come, which in our case involved deciding to transplant ourselves to a different continent: from suburban London to one of the small islands that lie scattered between Victoria and Vancouver in the Salish Sea, somewhat shielded from the Pacific Ocean.

Richard, half Canadian, had family on the West Coast. My own family was complicated and sometimes fraught. (It eventually became the basis of my novel *Dear Evelyn*.) I was one of three sisters, widely spaced in age: my eldest sister was seventeen years my senior and at sixteen had been mortified by the thought that if she pushed me in my pram, people would think I was hers. Our family began to scatter when I was still in elementary school, and my eldest sister and her husband immigrated to the USA. Now, my middle sister Jan (a mere twelve years my senior) and her husband were planning to follow their two daughters to New Zealand.

My relationship with my mother, difficult since adolescence, was still a challenge for both of us. The prospect of some distance did not alarm me. As for work, Richard would have space to set up a workshop and studio for the wooden furniture he intended to build to his own designs. I could write anywhere and pick up teaching work.

We did not realize quite how much we had to learn about the culture and history of the place we had moved to, and about ourselves too. But naive as we were, and as disastrous a move as this could have been, it worked out well. Along with much happiness, we have experienced the usual alarms, crises, losses, setbacks. Richard was eventually forced by some misshapen vertebrae and the demands of woodworking to abandon his custom furniture–making business and take on less satisfying work. He made the best of it, but I worried about him. Far from immune to fears and projections of disaster, I also worried about the education system, cellphones, children's screen time, and the internet. About teenage peer groups and sexuality. About windstorms, droughts, heating oceans, forest fires—the climate crisis predicted for half a century now real, right here, combined with a total lack of action from governments—of *that* I was and continue to be terrified. But I had no concerns about my own health or strength, which I continued until my early sixties to take completely for granted.

~

The beginning of a life-changing medical issue is frequently heralded by a fall, though I was ignorant of the matter of this when, in early April 2019, running downhill on a mountain trail, I tripped on a rock, lurched forwards and landed hard, breaking my fall with my right hand. This probably saved me from breaking my neck, but the wet cracking sound my hand made as it hit the rock did not bode well. I had fractured two fingers and mashed up the tissue, which understandably reacted with swelling, bruising, and pain.

Two doctors, one a hand specialist, warned the hand might take a year to *settle*. The hand troubles joined already long-standing pain in my right arm and shoulder (a complaint many writers develop) and worsened rather than improved. Despite physiotherapy, computer use grew increasingly difficult.

Never an athlete, I did enjoy keeping physically fit and appreciated its positive effects on my other activities. Now, in the wake of the fall, I had to suspend yoga and swimming, and I became a left-handed gardener, though I continued to hike and still sometimes jogged the easier trails.

It was disconcerting to note that my signature and handwriting, which had been fluid and large, became smaller, spikier, less controllable—*elderly* somehow. I had a busy year touring with a new novel and noticed it especially when signing books after readings. Naturally, I blamed the fall.

In February 2020—just before the Covid pandemic began—I was halfway up the same mountain, walking this time, when I developed an odd burning sensation in my chest. A heart attack? I knew women's symptoms could be milder, yet didn't think I was a likely candidate, and in any case, it quickly passed. A week later, after a few more such episodes, including one at home when merely sweeping the floor, Richard and I agreed that urgent action should be taken if it happened again.

He was beyond reach when it did recur. I drove to the emergency department. My doctor was on duty there and delivered the news: tests for cardiac markers showed elevated levels. I was to travel by ground ambulance and ferry to the cardiac unit in Victoria. She expressed her amazement at me of all people having such troubles. Since I'd not thought to bring any distractions, she kindly hurried to the staff room and returned with the novel she had in her bag.

The diagnosis was viral myocarditis (inflammation of the heart), *not* a heart attack, much better, even though my arteries were less perfect than I had assumed. Still, the recovery period was several months. I could go for walks but must not overtire myself. To prevent this, I'd been prescribed a beta blocker to "put the brakes on," as one physician said. I didn't like the effect, felt very apathetic and unlike myself. When I noticed a peculiar slowness in carrying out easy, ordinary tasks, I assumed it would go away when the medication stopped and my strength returned. My walking felt increasingly odd, too, tight and unnatural. Others began to notice. While walking, I was hyperaware of changes in surface and gradient, but after all, I reasoned, I had been through a lot.

A tremor began in my right hand and arm. Could it, too, be a side effect of medications I had been prescribed? This was one of several explanations offered online, another of which was Parkinson's disease.

"Drug-related is very unlikely," said the resident covering for my regular doctor. But I was delighted when she gave me permission to take a "medication vacation" to settle the matter. "I think this is an *intentional* tremor," she told me at the end of a very thorough masked appointment that included some neurological testing. Her eyes smiled as she spoke. I liked her. "Look. It's not there when your arm is relaxed. I would say this isn't the kind that comes with Parkinson's disease." Good news, I felt. On her return, my own doctor agreed.

"Though you can have both," a poet friend told me. "That happened with my dad."

~

That summer, to begin with rather cool, became unusually hot toward the end of August. The air thickened with the stench of forest fires in Washington and Oregon to the south of us, where thousands were fleeing their homes. The Arctic melted. Covid numbers surged. The rabid roar of right-wing mobs grew even louder, impossible to ignore. Ruth Bader Ginsburg died. Then the long, horrifying run-up to the US election. Conditions in my body seemed to be echoing the horrors out there in the world. But some things helped. It helped at night to lie warm and dry in bed next to the one I love, and by day to eat the garden's greens, beans, beets, squash, carrots; listen to its noisy birds, savour the sun, and gaze at yearning blue skies. To notice the many kinds of clouds. Mist. Rain. White rock and viridian conifer. The shimmering of rippled ocean, absolutely clear, pulled up tight over a pebble beach. Ravens calling to each other in flight. A mother deer and two speckled fawns. Meteors zipping across the inky sky.

In early autumn, Richard writes me a song. He and my son help me with newly difficult simple tasks. My sister, my best writer friend, and my editor phone regularly to check in and cheer me up— others call, or pick up, just at the right moment and don't mind settling in for the hour. I have long talks with kind strangers, the friends or acquaintances of friends, ready to offer information, contacts, ideas. Local friends seem happy to accommodate my new awkwardness and walk with me on the mountains, in the park, by the sea—always with trees nearby. Neighbours share a jellied treat, *birsalma sajt* (Hungarian), a.k.a. *membrillo* (Spanish), made from yellow quince; they bring jam, relish, brown bags of garden apples and perfect pears.

I'm given fitness programs, computer advice, osteopathic treatments. Bags of books and lists of titles to hunt down. A cashmere scarf in blues, greens, and pinks; another purple and gold; another light as air in dark subtle shades. Thoughtful emails, (terrible) jokes, and sudden tears. Paper letters folded inside hand-made cards. A thick woolen cardigan, a workbook on constructive thinking. I'm offered recommendations, advice, acknowledgment, encouragement, patience, and, where possible during a pandemic, real as well as virtual kisses.

Knowing that I am in others' thoughts—that I even appear in their dreams—warms and sustains me. And for me, there's *schadenfreude*'s sweet, lesser-known opposite, for which there is no German word. (*Freudenfreude*, invented by an American sociologist, is not actually German.) Fortunately, Sanskrit offers *mudita*: sympathetic joy, the pleasure that comes from delighting in other people's well-being.

And so, while symptoms do persist and worsen— and a tiny rusty-red blob smoulders where the sun should be in September's sky—I enjoy our son's happiness in his first-ever vehicle, an elderly orange-coloured truck. I'm happy because a formerly sad teacher friend of mine retired, took up wild swimming, and seems reborn. I think of a frustrated artist now building a studio in her garden, and of my widowed journalist neighbour giddily in love. Two other friends, a couple almost divorced, back together. One writer's risky eye surgery is safely completed; another's novel, eight years in the making, is finally being read and loved. Yet another has a story short-listed for a prize. Then there's my sister! Thriving and happy in New Zealand. My nephew did not die in the accident. His leg will heal. *Mudita, mudita!* Tell me your good news, I say, when people call. Bring it on. I'm not jealous. Don't be shy! I hoard such joys as if they were a bowl of the mottled pink and purple bean seeds from overgrown scarlet runners that my daughter used to call magic beans when she was little. I touch each in turn, feel the warmth of the sun that made them, and find solace in that same daughter, now twenty-four, and how she loves her new job—

But by the time October came around, it was clear to me that I did indeed have both kinds of tremor. I knew, too, that the odd slowness I was still experiencing had another name, *bradykinesia*, and was a well-known symptom of Parkinson's disease—and that faint, cramped handwriting, *micrographia*, was another. Everything to do with movement and coordination was rapidly getting worse; I was terrified, but as my doctor stressed, other explanations were still possible. It could be viral. It could be some kind of nerve damage from the fall. It could be MS, and that might show up on an MRI. Despite my doctor's efforts, I was still waiting for both the MRI and for an appointment with a neurologist. The speed with which I accrued new symptoms was apparently unusual, and no one was willing to actually diagnose me or prescribe anything other than antidepressants. But I had definitively crossed into the kingdom of the sick. I started taking the antidepressant and squared up to the wait.

That new grey passport brings new responsibilities. When you inhabit the kingdom of the sick, it is your job to understand, then explain your disease and the medical and bureaucratic systems it has forced you to be part of. You must learn a new vocabulary and teach it to those you love and those you are obliged to inform. Relaying to family, friends, and doctors the details and sensations of one's condition, along with various medical opinions, opaque test results, etc., not to speak of the emotional consequences of it all, is at times a huge relief. Yet it can soon become time-consuming and repetitive—doubtless for listeners, too, though of course there are those who care deeply, and others who have a curiosity about such things, as well as quite a few who enjoy the feeling of *schadenfreude*. (This last is merely an observation: I don't begrudge it them.)

Virginia Woolf, describing in "On Being Ill" "the undiscovered countries" of sickness, was frank about the impossibility, as she saw it, of understanding another's suffering. She noted: "Human beings do not go hand in hand the whole stretch of the way.

There is a virgin forest in each; a snowfield where even the print of birds' feet is unknown. Here we go alone, and like it better so." I love the prose but resist the final clause. Communication may be difficult and imperfect, yet I yearn and strive for it.

Even pre-Covid, when you could actually *be* with someone instead of seeing them on a blurry, freezing screen or just hearing their telephone voice, it was a challenge to fully enter into another person's lived physical reality. Separated from each other during lockdown, communication became more difficult. Add to that my ability to seem fairly coherent while actually falling apart, and misunderstanding is almost guaranteed. And of course, it is only natural that most listeners reach desperately for an experience of their own as comparison, though the malady may bear very little likeness other than that it concerns a physical dysfunction of some kind.

Still, it can feel wearing—even upsetting—to listen for forty-five minutes to a friend telling you of a miracle cure experienced for an entirely different ailment, or else relaying the details of a highly speculative, possibly-one-day-to-be-cutting-edge treatment for what you are experiencing, one that is unproven and not available to you for at least ten years and then only at enormous cost in another country. But remember: a citizen of the kingdom of the sick needs to develop patience and good manners.

The speaker means well. They, too, are in shock. Your news is unpleasant, and they want to offer something, to kindle hope, help in some way. What they are telling you is the best or first thing that came to mind. And somewhere, buried in it, may lie a nugget of useful information (or not). Remind yourself of this as your arm begins to shake from holding the phone. You will need your friends. Later, perhaps, you will learn how to take gentle control of such conversations.

Actually no, I have said many times, striving for a warm but authoritative tone, it's *not* my heart. That problem back in March was viral myocarditis, and that's all better. This is new. It's neurological. It's an as-yet-undiagnosed "movement disorder." Hands, arms, legs, muscles in general are affected, but it is actually rooted in my brain. I feel as if I am moving through water. As if I'm trying to drive a faulty machine. As if a spell has been cast over me. Nothing is ordinary or works as it should, and there is no ease or relief, except in sleep. I can't work; I'm on sick leave from the university . . . *No*, I'm not writing, and *yes*, I do know I must self-advocate and I do, zealously. But the system, underfunded, always slow, is now backed up due to the Covid-19 shutdown in the spring. Neurologists are scarce as snake hair, and sick people are everywhere, begging for attention. I can't fix those problems, and I have no idea when I will see a specialist or have a diagnosis but am told it will be months rather than weeks, probably not until next year.

Meanwhile, I take five minutes to tie my shoe-laces, then walk slower than I'd like to for an hour.

Judder my way through some recommended exercises every morning (effortful, slow). Try not to be utterly useless in the house. Eat—often with a spoon as it is easier. Answer email using occasionally hilarious error-prone dictation software. Talk to doctors and friends. Read. Time both creeps and rushes by.

If you can bear to take fair turns, the company of other sick people and attendant mutual commiseration can be very comforting. It can become overwhelming, so must be carefully done. My bookseller friend and I go back two decades; our same-age sons are still friends. We sit now in person (distanced) in the buttery autumn light to share our predicaments. I have delivered the full narrative of my fall and cascading symptoms; she now tells me the history of her hip troubles, which, we note, also began with a fall, in her case caused by stepping on an acorn.

An *acorn*? Yes. And yes, it's okay: she's smiling already. We might be able to laugh at this.

Leaving the organic food store with two heavy cloth bags, she trod on the acorn, which then rolled beneath her foot. Initially this tipped her backwards. Instinct told her not to go that way and dash the back of her head on the pavement. She swung her arms forward—each laden with a heavy cloth bag—briefly righted herself, then crashed onto her hands and knees. Apples, carrots, and potatoes spilled from her bags.

Her right knee and hip absorbed most of the impact. Both grew more painful in the ensuing weeks. Sitting, standing, and turning became a set of inescapable agonies. During this time, her husband decided to leave her, though later he changed his mind.

Thirteen months on, she's diagnosed with internal derangement. A muscle has slipped out of place and can only be fixed by risky surgery.

We two fallen women eat a bowl of just-picked plums and laugh about internal derangement. Deranged is something we both feel right now. We compare it to my intentional tremor, which sounds to the uninitiated as if I'm shaking on purpose, a thing that could not be further from the truth. We agree that the tremor at rest I also have seems like a contradiction in terms and speculate as to the possibility of *intentional derangement*.

It's extraordinarily good to be able to laugh about being sick.

Making comparisons is potentially dangerous—but we risk it and agree, after some debate, that my condition is likely worse than hers, nasty as that is. Both are disabling, but mine seems likely to be *progressive* (another strange and appalling word, given the meaning is that it inexorably gets worse), incurable, and life-abbreviating. This may make her feel relatively fortunate; I don't ask.

After my friend's visit, I remember something that predates my own fall by several years and may be evidence of the real beginning of what is happening to me.

I'd set a pan of rice to cook. Sitting not far away, I was soon absorbed in editing some short stories and only eventually looked up and *saw* smoke; I smelled nothing, even though the pan had burnt to black at the bottom. Extensive tests ruled out a brain tumour and various other possibilities; a specialist diagnosed rhinitis.

She did not mention, though, that loss of the sense of smell, *anosmia*, can be an early sign of Parkinson's disease. Later, the information came up online, but I had no other symptoms and it seemed unlikely. I'd put the knowledge aside and—fortunately, I feel, since nothing could have been done at that point—forgotten it.

Life—teaching, writing, family, garden—was busy on all fronts. I biked, hiked, and swam. Just six months before my fall, I'd completed a hiking tour at altitude in Peru. I chaired the Creative Writing department, published a new book of stories, my eighth novel . . .

"Do you think my loss of smell could be significant?" I asked my doctor during the next phone appointment.

"It could be," she said, "but the neurologist will be the best person to answer that."

"The unattainable neurologist."

She joined me in a brittle little laugh.

Anxious, unable to sleep, I lie on my back in the inky dark and think of my family and friends. What can I do for them? Often the answer is not very much at all—but even the smallest thing feels good. One writer friend recommends a book called *How to Do Nothing*. I joke that I am doing it rather well. You sound too stoical, she says.

Stoical? If so, it's a public face. On my own, at home, it's different. Tears streamed down my face when my doctor suggested on the phone that my symptoms might be virally induced and so there was at least a chance that they might therefore resolve, given time.

These were tears of sheer gratitude at the possibility of getting better, of release from one story into another somewhat, possibly better one. Later, Richard and I cried together when we admitted to ourselves that "the golden virus" idea was a mirage. And then I cried alone in the woods, thinking how much my relationship with him has changed and will change, how it is becoming one where he helps and looks after me more than formerly and I am no longer a powerful equal in our life together, but a dependent. I cried for both of us. I asked him would he need someone else more functional to keep him sane. No, he said, of course not. More tears.

I sobbed when I felt alone with all the unpleasant information I was acquiring and hoarding so as to avoid overwhelming those close to me. Most recently, I howled when I could not do a simple piece of foot and arm coordination during an online exercise class—it was a small aggravation that stood in for everything—I wailed, doubled over in the face of this momentary humiliation, in the face of my new powerlessness, of all the many losses. There was rage, fear, and desperation. Richard came to comfort me; our son, three rooms away and wearing headphones to participate in an online seminar, heard nothing. It felt good to cry without restraint.

I'm no stoic, but you can't be howling all the time.

~

I am lucky to have any financial support at all, but who would have thought that not being at work would be so much work? Leaflets, emails, letters, forms. Insurance-speak. The bureaucracy of sickness:

> You have responsibilities that are key to the management of your claim. It is expected that you will make reasonable efforts to participate in reasonable treatment and rehabilitation, advise us of any changes in your condition, work towards returning to your own occupation, or assist in identifying other suitable employment, and/or accept reasonable offers of alternate or modified work from your employer.

I note three *reasonable*s in one sentence, along with a single *suitable*, but this is not for me to point out.

It's important to remember that people who ask, "But are you doing *your own work*?," meaning writing, are just trying to understand. But the question does seem preposterous. They are asking whether, despite being mysteriously, multiply dysfunctional to the point of being unable to sustain half a teaching load at the university, I am somehow capable of functioning as a novelist, i.e., doing one of the most exciting but also most mentally and even physically demanding things there is, along with associated administrative and publicizing tasks.

Novel writing can be playful and fun, but whether you are the planning sort or you write into a void to find out what the story might be, it is one of the most mentally demanding activities there is. You must develop your characters along with their background and backstory (which may scarcely appear, but nonetheless powerfully informs the material you do use). You need to know and understand their desires, fears, and contradictions and their relationships to those they are involved with and their wider community—use all those to generate the narrative, at some point find the best point of view, the beginning, the way to end, the pace at which to build and reveal the story, and how to include the subplots. You also need to remember or settle on where you are going and sustain a sense of the book's overall shape, its structure. You must imagine the sentence-by-sentence experience of a hypothetical reader. All this, not to speak of revision and editing, takes brainwork, both creative and organizational, on a grand scale. Brainwork is demanding physically. Haruki Murakami, in *What I*

Talk About When I Talk About Running, equates finishing a novel with running marathons and manual labour. He says that "a writer puts on an outfit called narrative and thinks with his entire being; and for the novelist that process requires putting into play all your physical reserve."

It's painful to explain over and over that it takes me at least four times as long as normal simply to clean my teeth or get my pants on. That I need to *think through* how to turn a T-shirt the right way out and put the correct but mysteriously juddering and trembling arm through the appropriate sleeve, and so perhaps it is not surprising that, leaving aside my current lack of energy and ideas, I'm unable to write normally even in the purely mechanical sense, let alone expend all the mental and physical energy a novel or even a short story requires.

I do miss working with words. *If* I had an idea in my head, maybe I could write a haiku now and then, or a page-long moment story in a month or two. I'd be happy to manage either of these. Meanwhile, I jot my observations in dreadful, tremulous handwriting in a notebook. When—if—I'm able, I hope to find a way to put these observations together, a few lines at a time, and make them into something; I'm not sure what, but thinking this way does allow me to recreate for myself a sense of agency and to separate some part of myself from my predicament.

There's surely more than a whiff of residual romanticism behind the notion that my normal kind of "own work" might be possible when I'm falling apart—a belief that a real writer will and should be driven, no matter what, to use their last ounce of energy to write. I understand that my friends see writing novels as fundamental to my identity. Until recently I felt that way, too, but very quickly, like any new citizen here in the other place, I have been forced to imagine otherwise, and to renegotiate the possible.

In the new year, there is a cold ferry ride and then a long drive through rain and mist to a down-at-heel clinic in a half-deserted mall. The receptionist warns that the doctor always runs late, and he does, by almost an hour. But I don't care. It's a real face-to-face appointment that I have waited nine months for. And this doctor I'm to see is not actually a neurologist but a gerontologist amply qualified to assess me.

He's a short, smallish man, middle-aged. We're both medically masked, of course, he at his desk in a corner facing the wall and I seated so that I see him from the side. Exhibiting several of them as I do so, I catalogue my symptoms as calmly and economically as possible. He studies the referral letter intently as I speak, yet he somehow listens. Eventually, he examines me, puts me through some tests, and then, to my surprise, helps me get my shoes back on prior to a walk down the corridor and back.

"You do have several symptoms of Parkinson's disease," he confirms as he settles back into his chair. "Your walking, tremors, and slowness are the most noticeable." He advises that the best next step is to take a medication called carbidopa/levodopa. If it works, and he thinks it will, the diagnosis will be confirmed. He writes a blood-work requisition and a prescription: I should take a slowly increasing dose over a month or so to determine the appropriate amount and then continue for another two months to see how stable my response is and whether any side effects are tolerable.

Like many people, I have heard about levodopa because Oliver Sacks wrote about it in his extraordinary book, later made into a movie, *Awakenings*. An epidemic of encephalitis lethargica, or "sleepy sickness," infected thousands of people worldwide in the 1920s, leaving many with permanent, very severe Parkinson's-like symptoms. Largely immobile, dazed, and seemingly apathetic, these survivors were cared for over decades in dedicated wards and institutions.

By Sacks's time, it was understood that dopamine, a neurohormone and a neurotransmitter produced in several places in the brain, and informally known as a chemical messenger, is vital to the function of many organs and bodily systems, including but far from limited to movement, cognition, and mood. Many Parkinson's symptoms are caused by a lack of it.

When, in 1969, the price of a new dopamine replacement drug called levodopa, or L-DOPA, became affordable, Sacks prescribed it to a group of eighty encephalitis lethargica patients who had existed in a kind of spellbound condition for four decades inside the New York hospital where he was working at the time.

The effect varied from patient to patient but often was swift and quasi-miraculous, with patients quickly waking from their long somnolence to experience the joys of movement and communication. During the preceding decades, they had apparently been aware of their environment and situation, yet unable or unmotivated to respond; now life could begin again. In a 1985 interview on NPR, Sacks described witnessing this transformation as "like seeing frozen figures thawing. And with this, a great delight as an awakening or sort of resurrection might be expected to have."

But amazing as the results were, problems soon developed. Awake, and sometimes even hyperalert, the patients were in many ways still the young people they had been when they became lethargic; since that point, they'd had no new experiences, missed out on normal life, and formed very few new memories. They had not really matured emotionally or intellectually as they aged. Many were without family or friends. As well as that, the drug, given then at a high dose, had inconsistencies and unwanted effects which many found intolerable. Very few of the patient stories shared by Sacks have happy endings, though some do.

The use of levodopa has been somewhat refined since *Awakenings* was written, but the treatment for Parkinson's has, like Sacks's lethargic patients, been in a static state for many years. The same synthetic dopamine precursor is still the main drug prescribed, though it is now often combined with carbidopa, an enhancement that prevents levodopa from being broken down before it crosses the blood-brain barrier and is made into usable dopamine. The benefits of this are that some of the unwanted side effects may be slower to appear and the dose of levodopa can be smaller. This is important. Although the initial effect of dopamine replacement on a Parkinson's patient can be miraculous, as the disease progresses and as higher and more frequent doses are required, for most people the drug becomes increasingly problematic.

Toward the end of the consultation, feeling oddly calm, I call Richard into the consulting room and provide a précis.

"I won't hold you to it, but how long do you think it will work for me?" I ask the oddly unexpressive and yet, I feel, deeply compassionate doctor.

"Everyone is different—" He meets my gaze for what seems like the first time. "It's useful for ... *a number* of years. Typically, between six and fifteen. I will say, though, that your symptoms seem to have been developing quickly rather than slowly."

He hands me the prescription and the requisition for blood work.

"It's very hard to know what to do," Richard says. "We need to downsize. I'd like to get our ducks in a row, but—"

"I wouldn't advise you to make any big decisions until we've done this trial. I'll see you again late April," the doctor tells us, closing the file on his desk as he does so. "Hopefully after that, you'll have an appointment with Neurology."

"If I need to, may I ask questions on the phone?"

"I'll try to respond," he says. "But I'm busy. As you saw, I always run late." I thank him profusely for fitting me in, a kindness I won't forget.

In the seating area beyond the consulting room, other patients sit waiting, spaced apart, masked, eyes glazed. Outside, the mist has turned to rain; concrete, asphalt, and sky are darkening their greys.

"How do you feel?" Richard asks once we are in the car.

"Hungry," I tell him, struggling to remove the lid from the jar of nuts we brought with us. "I'm not delighted," I tell him. And certainly, I could be feeling better (Doc said he's seen this before, and it passes), or I could be feeling worse (if, say, he'd thought that I have multiple system atrophy or supranuclear palsy). "He gave the impression he's pretty sure I have Parkinson's, and I don't want to have it. But we suspected it anyway, and being seen, being spoken to honestly, and given some kind of potential treatment, it's at least a step forward. Better than limbo. Verging on positive."

"Yes," my sweet husband says, and he starts the car, turns on the fan. The windshield is fogged up, and the rain—noisy now—falls thick and fast. "That's pretty much it."

Half a yellow pill three times a day is intended to connect your body with the drug and to expose any unwelcome effects. It's not expected to be enough. Even so, something happens. The effects are subtle yet definitely present: the tremor is subdued, if still lurking. Steadier hands, a greater feeling of physical calmness. Perhaps my walking is a little better? Some things seem somewhat easier to do, others not— there's a taste of honey, at least. At the end of ten days, I double the dose and within the day comes real sweetness. To begin with, I hardly dare to speak of it, and in any case, how can I describe this loosening of my bonds to someone who has not suffered months of restriction and feeling bewitched?

I'm moving more freely, walking almost normally. Everything's easier, but far more than that—everything is a pleasure. Imagine: Taking the stairs two at a time. Reaching to the high shelf. Opening a door. Almost slamming it. Pouring water from a jug. Holding a full cup in one hand. Emptying the dishwasher: swoop down—up—reach—twist—slot plates in the rack. And all without being continuously aware that I used to do this better and something terrible is wrong with me.

Ordinary movements are a kind of dance—and who cares that dancing is something I've never been good at? This is it, here I am!

I feel as if I have sneaked back across the border into the kingdom of the well. I slip my arms at an almost normal pace into my jacket, zip it up on only the second attempt, competently tie my shoelaces in a matter of seconds, then stride out into the world. Yes, I do still have to remind myself to swing my arms, but less often than before; they swing higher and faster, and neither hand is twitching, not at all. I walk down-hill, uphill, on the flat; I walk fast and hard and savour every step, sometimes breaking into a skip or a jog. When my artist friend and I are hiking and reach the lookout point just before the summit of the moun-tain, it is ice and snow on the trail, not my fatigue, that prevent us from continuing to the top. I'm cer-tain we'll get there next week. Meanwhile, wind combs our hair as we absorb the silvery sea, the pro-fusion of islands, the infinite hues of a blue-grey sky.

Because my body is moving more freely and does not claim my attention, my mind is liberated too. I notice and think about things other than my own sensations and situation. Anything. Everything. It's all there. As Sacks puts it in *Awakenings*, albeit writ-ing about patients far deeper into their disease than I have yet travelled in mine:

> The awakened patient . . . falls in love with
> reality itself. . . . Where, previously, he felt ill

at ease, uncomfortable, unnatural, and strained, he now feels at ease, and at one with the world. All aspects of his being—his movements, his perceptions, his thoughts, and his feelings—testify simultaneously to the fact of awakening. The stream of being, no longer clogged or congealed, flows with an effortless, unforced ease . . . There is a great sense of spaciousness, of freedom of being. The instabilities and knife-edges of disease disappear, and are replaced by poise, resilience, and ease.

(I'm aware that *ease* is used four times, but it is a lovely word.) These feelings, as Sacks so aptly writes, "show us the full quality—the zenith of real being (so rarely experienced by most 'healthy' people); they show us what we have known—and almost forgotten; what all of us once had—and have subsequently lost."

I have reread this book; I've studied the ongoing research online. I know that my visa is a temporary one, that this current bliss won't last forever, but I refuse to dwell on that, except to note that right now impermanence makes its flavour yet more complex and intense.

"If only we could have a party!" I tell my husband and kiss him on the neck as he touches fingers to keys—not knowing, as I now do, that to do so is a miracle—and makes words appear on a screen.

2

~

Kitchen Dance

Richard, slightly drunk, loads the dishwasher, while I lean against the kitchen counter savouring the last of my bowl of ice cream. I am two months into treatment, and being able to make dinner—rapid chopping involving good coordination of left and right hands, unscrewing jars, lifting of heavy pans, all that mundanity—still seems miraculous. Just a stir-fry and noodles, but so good. Richard reaches for a soy-smeared plate, stops just before picking it up, straightens, turns to face me.

"Oh, I'm sorry!" he says, rubbing his hands on the sides of his jeans. "I've really let myself go." *Let go?* Since he's clearly so unhappy, I know he's referring to self-neglect rather than release from inhibition.

"You look lovely," I tell him. A reflex, but sincere. "What is this?"

"I'm putting on weight again!" he says. I've not noticed it. He is of course growing older, but not nearly so fast as I am. He's aging at a normal pace in that interesting, characterful way that some mange to achieve, especially if they remain emotionally and intellectually open to the world. He's not turned into a cartoon character, fossilized into one version of himself as so many do. Inside, he has ripened. As for the exterior, his warm, curious gaze is unchanged, even though his hazel eyes look out from a face more deeply carved into its familiar planes. His hair fades evenly from iron lower down to silver on top; he tends more often to stubble, which may suggest underlying changes to the jaw, but his full, generous lips are unchanged. He's troubled by various aches and pains. Who is not?

"I don't know how it happened." He slips a plate carefully into its groove in the rack, stands, turns again to face me. He's near to tears! His voice wavers. "I want you to know I intend to tackle it."

"Oh, don't beat yourself up—" I begin. And then we're in each other's arms. Maybe there *is* a little more of him than there used to be, but what I am aware of is the warm, live feeling of his flesh, and how well I know and love the body he's currently at odds with. How I would like to spend more time pressed together like this.

Richard has always been particular about how he looks and prone to sudden, and often ineffective, diets. I was periodically anorexic until my twenties and have at times been similarly prone, though perhaps less extreme and more scientific about it, as well as becoming year by year less able to sustain the concern. One way or another, since we met and shared our lives with each other, we've both gladly relinquished our residual fanaticism in respect of body image. But of course, aesthetics and appetite aren't what matter here. They are the very least of it, a mere carrier for larger concerns.

I feel that Richard is overwhelmed by how many important things (my health, the pandemic, the climate) are unravelling. Perhaps his middle-aged body, emblematic for him of these fears and anxieties, seems like something he might possibly be able to control in a world where other far more important things are well beyond his influence—just as my adolescent body seemed for me all those years ago?

Not long before this moment in our kitchen, when my symptoms were at their untreated worst, I experienced an inverted version of the same crisis. Submerged in weakness and dysfunction, acutely aware of the unnerving judders and tremors and the unsettling sense of precarious balance that what I used to think of as *my* body delivered on a continuous basis, I knew that I also *looked* terrible: that is, more than half dead. It was frightening, so I did my best to avoid protracted exposure to the suddenly nonagenarian face that glared back at me from the mirror when I brushed my thinning hair or made my best effort in terms of dental hygiene. Deep lines. Jowls. Weary, waxy skin. Simultaneously vanishing and unruly eyebrows; a moustache, mostly blonde.

Worst of all, newly asymmetrical eyes, the right one hooded and slanting, the left fully open much as it used to be, both equally involved in an angry, terrified glare that I found repellent yet could only alter briefly by vigorously feigning mirth.

I had plenty of other problems and found it easy not to dwell on my appearance. But one evening, I mistakenly removed and hung up my towel before emerging from the bathroom and was confronted in the long mirror opposite the door with a horrifying vision of the whole new me. Boney and narrow, I was clearly still losing weight, despite my voracious appetite. Tendons stood out on my neck. I already knew my breasts had shrunk, but now I saw that they were *withered*: deep creases ran like rays to the nipples. Piano key ribs. Jutting hips. Arms that had lost most of their muscle. Veins snaked up these weak-looking limbs, and likewise my legs, also ghosts of their former sturdy selves. Above the greying pubic hair and ancient C-section scar, someone had tossed a net of blue veins over my abdomen. My poor husband! I tended to keep covered up, but should he catch sight of me this way, it would be like climbing into bed with a medieval memento mori.

The mirror's image did not merely reflect and remind me of how I felt inside. The reflection amplified it. Panic-stricken, I tugged a T-shirt from the drawer, fought my way into it.

Beneath the revulsion, pity and compassion lurked, yet why care? It seemed like a colossal waste of time and energy to dwell on my body's appearance—so much less important than its functioning and the sensations it inflicted.

Mindfulness instructors and yoga teachers often stress the importance of connecting with one's body, being aware of it, *in* it, rather than chasing thoughts and daydreams and forgetting it exists. Why, though, would I want to be *in my body*, given that, due to malfunction in the part of it called the brain, it gives me such grief? The various pains. The involuntary clenching of some muscles, the rigidity of others. Pain. Constant fatigue, a peculiar gait, dizziness, fumbling fingers: these are the things I wish to escape rather than inhabit.

As many have before me, I feel I am my body's prisoner. Or, for variety, that I am a harried driver on an empty road many miles away from home, strapped into a faulty machine, a vehicle jinxed by an ever-growing list of malfunctioning parts only some of which can be temporarily patched up and all of which will eventually combine into a hair-raising downhill skid toward a precipice.

Given the nature of our society, it's no surprise that we often speak of our bodies as possessions—important but ultimately inferior owned things, like vehicles, that come in basic or more luxurious, status-conveying variations.

Driver and vehicle, boss and worker—pretty much every image that springs up when considering our relationship with our physicality suggests that there is a separate self-mind-soul, some kind of mental or spiritual superior entity, emanating from or created by the grey matter in our skulls—often felt to be situated just behind our foreheads, in the middle, looking out as it absorbs, reflects, makes choices, and all the while tries to care for and control the thoughtless, inchoate raw thing that supports it.

To some extent, neuroscience confirms this feeling: the prefrontal cortex which orchestrates the high-level decision-making known as executive function is indeed housed at the front of the brain, in the middle of and behind of the forehead. It's not however considered a separate entity, like an organ, but more a site of activity, connected to many other parts of brain.

Strict boundaries seem to be out of fashion. Some now think that humans may be ecologies or cultures rather than discrete beings, as research has discovered that the human cells we are born with are gradually outnumbered by the microbes living on and inside us.

In any case, flesh is determined to ultimately become unreliable, painful, inefficient. At some point, all our remedies, procedures, medicines, exercise routines, diets, surgeries, prayers, rituals, and precautions fail. As muscle, bone, organs, nerve, and even sentience itself become burdensome, and attempts to control the obstinately dysfunctional mass of organic systems bring diminishing success, many seek to distance their supposedly higher-value selves from brute physicality. It's no longer *my* body but *this* body, then *this + expletive of choice* body or body part.

These days, I can walk past that long mirror naked or dressed in my too-loose, out-of-style clothes and see a changed woman, graceless, awkward, and ungainly, prematurely *old*, for sure, but distinctive and even somehow interesting, to me at least. There are stories there, struggle, and doubtless more damage to come. This thing I'm in (or that we are, human and bacteria together) is still prepared to do its best. For now, at least, I'm grateful for its willingness and persistence.

Disembodied existence is currently impossible. While the brain part of the body contains information and neural pathways particular to the person we are, it, too, is biological, fleshy, and, as yet, mortal. Brain and body, inextricably linked, would do well to love each other, but this seems hard to achieve and sustain.

In the kitchen Richard and I, who do without effort love one another, engage in a strange, staggering, welded-together dance, the two of us pressed into one asymmetrical shape. We come to a halt in the middle of the room. I squeeze him to me as tightly as I can. I'm stronger than I have been for a long while. My arms have grown a little bit of muscle; my legs look almost normal. The breast creases are on the way out. I've gained some pounds. It's mainly down to the medication, but I'm proud of my cells, biome, and whatever else might be involved for taking advantage of the opportunity.

"We don't stay the same," I mutter into the damp heat of my husband's shoulder, and for a moment or two, I find the thought almost exciting, a kind of liberation. *I will love you however you are*, I think but do not say aloud. *Whoever I am, and whatever I become.* I like it. If we got married again, perhaps we could use those words instead of *in sickness and health.*

3

~

The Man in the Red-Light Hat

I t's my first time at the support group. Rob's wife, Eliza, invited me.

Nigel and Pam, also new, look to be the youngest attendees: mid-fifties, perhaps. She, artistic and willowy, swathed in jewel-coloured, flowing clothes, smiles often and nods benevolently (or is it royally?) as others speak; he, soft-spoken, elf-like, was only recently diagnosed. He distrusts the offered medications and the mainstream medical system in general and so is exploring alternatives—such as the red-light hat he has brought with him to demonstrate. This device looks somewhat like a cycling helmet, and he clips it beneath his chin in just the same way. It's made of plastic strips arranged in a honeycomb shape and studded inside with bulbs that emit both red light and near-infrared (NIR) light in a combination said to have positive, even regenerative effects on the brain. The honeycombing is for ventilation.

With a flourish, Nigel taps the switch. Bursts of red light flutter and pulse in the helmet, creating some interesting effects on his face. Similar light therapy helmets sell for thousands, he tells us, but this is a much cheaper homemade version, put together from a plan that he downloaded from the internet. He wears it for twenty minutes a day. Lightweight and very comfortable, he says. You forget you have it on!

Can he feel anything inside his head while it's working? I imagine a fizzing feeling, a tingling, a tickling—

No. But he feels better afterwards.

Does the light penetrate Nigel's skull and reach deep into his midbrain where the neurons are damaged and dying?

NIR light does pass through bone, he says, though it might not travel so far as the ailing and dying neurons in the substantia nigra, that small, murky midbrain region that helps control the body's movement and plays a role in mood, judgment, and other processes affected by Parkinson's. But it's very beneficial for other brain cells that may, in ways not yet understood, be protective or even supportive of neural regeneration.

Later, I check. NIR and red light: different but related. NIR is the more penetrating, but you may as well have both. Photobiomodulation. Mitochondria. Schwann cells. Wavelength. Intensity. Reduced inflammation. It's complicated, yes, but not crazy. I remind myself that red light therapies being very much in vogue with healthy people seeking longevity and younger-looking skin is not a reason to dismiss it. Research is in the early stages.

In a 2019 study, Nigel tells us, six Parkinson's patients spent time in a helmet like his every day. They reported improved facial expression, auditory processing, engagement in conversation, sleep quality, and motivation. There is word of another ongoing study of 120 patients using a more sophisticated helmet.

In 2020, a different seven patients had a fibre optic cable implanted right into their brains to deliver pulses of NIR light directly to the substantia nigra. Results are eagerly awaited. Meanwhile, Nigel feels his device is working for him. I later learn that two other members of the group have similar hats.

NIR is still experimental. Deep brain stimulation (DBS), once way out on the fringes, is now mainstream and fully embraced by the medical profession, even though how it works is still unclear. It involves drilling holes in the skull to implant electrodes in the brain, and another minor surgery to implant a battery-containing device under the skin of the chest or neck. The user then adjusts the stimulation using a hand-held device rather like a cellphone. DIY in this instance is not recommended.

DBS surgeons are rare where I live, but the treatment is just about available in a not-too-distant hospital to a small number of suitable patients who have survived the wait-list without degenerating to the point that it would not work for them.

It's only recommended for some PWP (people with Parkinson's), and there is an elaborate screening process. Adjusting the stimulation is a fine art. Too much of it negatively affects speech, may cause double vision, balance and mood problems. But mostly it's good news. Users speak of having their lives turned around.

Nigel, still crowned with the helmet of flashing red, continues in a gentle, even tone to share some information about his research into possible causes of the disease, as well as his diet, exercise, and meditation routines—which, he points out, pulling a quick smile, pretty much amount to a full-time job. With a flourish, he removes his headgear, switches it off, and suddenly becomes ordinary again.

"Hard act to follow!" someone says amidst a gentle smattering of applause.

A support group offers companionship, information sharing. Listening. Though, of course, it is a big step to take: that was how Eliza expressed it when she invited me, *big step* meaning a further, deeper level of acknowledgment of this disease in me. And recognition that the group will confront me with a variety of more *progressed* (translation: awful) futures, some of which may be mine.

"You could wait. Save it for when you're worse," one friend suggested after I told her I might attend.

When. "You already seem well-informed and have supportive friends," she pointed out. True.

But, curious by nature, I'm keen to make my understanding less abstract. To see for myself what the new words I am learning refer to in life beyond the page or pamphlet, what they *mean* in actual life. And after all, I thought, perhaps disingenuously, I can just test the group out. So I accepted Eliza's invitation, and then others too. In the course of a few months, I met more people than I have in entire years.

Men predominate. Fair enough, given incidence is three times as high for male PWP. However, they are frequently accompanied by female care partners, some of whom, utterly exhausted, look far sicker than their spouses. Margaret, her hair thinning, her entire body, every pouch and pocket of flesh, utterly weary, explains in an oddly cheery tone that her husband won't use his walker or sticks and so keeps falling when they go out together; he is too heavy for her to lift and in any case will not accept help. She must leave him to struggle to his feet in the middle of the mall or street and explain repeatedly to concerned bystanders why she is not assisting him.

She shrugs, grins, looks around at us bright-eyed, as if the most outrageous joke had just been told. At any moment, I feel, she might implode.

He, motionless next to her, stares angrily ahead.

No one knows what to say.

The carers need their own group (and a lot else besides) is what I think but don't dare to articulate.

(I learn later that there used to be one, but it's not yet been revived following Covid restrictions.) A silence grows, and then Eliza says, very quietly in just the right tone of voice, "It's all so difficult."

The only male care partner present today is Caroline's husband. Now and then, he gently corrects her or adds supplementary information. At one point, he takes her hand between his. A small, good thing to cling to is that adversity does generate kindness, in some at least.

Pearl lives alone. She worries night and day about how and where she will go when she can't manage her already-too-large home and who, when it comes to it, will look after her. How much will that cost? But Valerie, formerly a pianist, describes the enviably slow fifteen-year progression of her disease as "like watching paint dry" and shares that she has begun and is enjoying singing lessons—something she never got around to when she was well. There seem to be no negatives at all! Though she does admit to finding dental hygiene difficult; the motivation, she says, as much as anything. Her dry wit is bracing. There's not a great deal of panache or exuberance in these groups.

People speak quietly. It is easily forgotten that pretty much every bit and type of musculature can be affected by Parkinson's, including the small but crucial muscles in the throat and mouth. They lose strength and coordination. Inflection is dampened, the voice becomes soft, slurred, tremulous. At the same time, the brain's audio feedback mechanism may decline, so the speaker does not realize how quiet or flat their speech has become and misses the chance to correct it. Throw in the frustration of forgetting what you wanted to say, and for some the effort seems disproportionate to the outcome.

Swallowing and speech disorders eventually afflict most of us. Realizing you speak in a flat monotone and have become hard to understand is horrible, especially for those whose work depends on skilled use of their voices. Humiliation, shame, anxiety, and a reluctance to socialize only confound the problem. Speech therapy and technological aids are helpful, but wait-lists are long and how much one can benefit from these often depends on ability to pay.

Being unable to talk is one of my worst nightmares.

Years ago, severe laryngitis stole my voice for several weeks. I communicated via notes and soon noticed that people tended to answer my paragraph-long messages simply and quickly, even, as time passed, monosyllabically or with a simple gesture. Over time, I tended to only say simple things. It was nothing like conversation. It was hard for people to converse with me when doing something else, as so often happens in life. Even my own loving family unwittingly treated me like a ghost—until my tween-aged daughter thought to reply in note form rather than speech, thus equalizing us. Later, at university, she learned sign language and sometimes uses it in her work, but I don't think that would be of great service for this group.

"Bits of your life are constantly plucked away," Tony says, and with his next breath affirms his enduring belief in God's benevolence. Another man's wife lost her sight at the same time as his diagnosis, so they have been unable to look after each other as they wish. Another's diagnosis took almost a decade and was only resolved when his irritable and baffled GP sent him to a psychiatrist, who immediately picked up on his cramped handwriting.

Some seem welded to their chairs; others stand rather than sit, the better to accommodate back problems or various kinds of involuntary movements. These jerks, writhing, nods, bobs, and bows are often more distressing to others than to the person in motion, who cares more about pain level, mobility, and how alert and functional they feel than about how they may seem to others. About what they can still *do*.

Given the legion of symptoms, how horrible they are, the way they accumulate, and the finite nature of the relief granted by the yellow pills, we're bound to seek alternatives, dream of actual cures, and fundraise or donate to get the research done. As for trying the unproven, some are braver than others, or richer, or both—but everyone is interested. Along with comparisons and suggestions about drug regimens, news of alternative or experimental treatments, of promising discoveries and medical trials features largely at meetings.

Vibrating gloves. Could you wear them at the same time as the helmet?

Terazosin: highly recommended by another writer. Most doctors will not prescribe terazosin other than for its original purposes, the treatment of high blood pressure or of prostate disease; its other effect came to light by accident. Of a group of thirty thousand men with Parkinson's, the fifteen hundred who were taking the alpha-blocker for their inflamed prostrates were found either to be not progressing (remember, that means worsening) or progressing more slowly. Off-label uses of terazosin have not been properly studied. It can produce negative, even fatal, side effects, but since Parkinson's has nasty effects, too, some are keen to experiment.

But what about a nice and natural remedy you can grow yourself? Fava beans contain both levodopa and carbidopa! That said, much of it is in the pods rather than the beans, and it is impossible to eat enough of them to have an effect without bursting.

Grown in hot climates and recommended both as an aphrodisiac and for those hoping to reduce body fat, the velvet bean, *Mucuna pruriens*, contains 6 to 9 percent levodopa by weight, but no carbidopa, which may negatively affect absorption. A woman in the support group is trying velvet beans in powdered form but still has the same problems with her legs.

Rob is taking vitamin B1 at a very high dose plus vitamin B12. Vitamin B6, on the other hand, may negatively affect the absorption of L-DOPA, but only if that L-DOPA is not mixed with carbidopa . . .

Fecal transplant! Yes. Since Parkinsonian guts harbour a distinctly destructive population of bacteria, fungi, and so on, and the connection between gut biome and brain health is established, there's hope that a fecal transplant from someone with a healthier biome might treat motor symptoms as well as constipation and depression. The transplant is achieved by enema or capsules. One donation (apparently it's processed to extract the microbes) serves three recipients.

Squeamish? Probiotics may do some of the same things, though only certain very expensive strains.

Could a spoonful a day of mannitol keep brain rot at bay? Found in many plants and widely used as a food sweetener, this substance may inhibit the misfolding and clumping of alpha-synuclein proteins that kill dopamine-producing brain cells. Also, it is known to make the blood-brain barrier more permeable, so it may increase the absorption of L-DOPA. Neither efficacy nor safety at the dose suggested are proven, but reported side effects are not too bad: gas, diarrhea.

CBD (cannabidiol) might help with sleep but may leave you feeling not so sharp when awake and could interact with other medications. Legal (here) but not necessarily approved of by your neurologist (if you have one).

Microdoses of psilocybin, derived from magic mushrooms. The new panacea! Legalization may eventually occur.

Ibogaine, derived from a shrub that grows in Western Equatorial Africa, is traditionally used in initiation and other ceremonies, as well as a remedy for fever and (again) an aphrodisiac. Handy! Due to its reported ability to treat addiction, there has been some research into it. Ibogaine increases the production of a protein called glial cell line-derived neurotrophic factor, or GDNF, which may be neuroprotective and, some suggest, possibly act to *restore* function in damaged dopamine neurons, or even create new ones. Outliers trying it at a microdose level for Parkinson's report positively—though, of course, in this case and in all cases, there is a very powerful placebo effect to take into account.

In the first chapter of *Cured: A Journey into the Science of Mind over Body*, Jo Marchant explores some experiments and investigations into the way placebo works, including research by Dr. Jon Stoessl of the University of British Columbia, who used brain scans to show that after taking an "empty" placebo pill, participants felt as if they had taken their real drug, and this had a basis in what was actually happening in the brain. Marchant concludes that while there are "crucial limitations . . . the effects of placebos are underpinned by measurable, physical changes in the brain and body."

Like terazosin, ibogaine can have serious, even fatal, side effects which would be a cause for concern even if beneficial effects were proven. In any case, it's no longer legally obtainable in Canada, a shame since it's the one I'm most drawn to . . . along with the red-light helmet. And stem cells (not yet available for PWP).

Despite the group's interest in these topics, I don't think many people go further than eating more vegetables and buying a supplement or two.

"How far would you go for an experimental treatment?" my sister Jan asks me during a discussion of stem cell therapy. She lives in New Zealand and successfully used it there to treat her arthritic joints. I tell her about Hal, who travelled against the advice of his doctors to Ukraine (pre-war) to obtain an early form of stem cell treatment for Parkinson's. Currently in the "doing very well" category, he says he has no idea whether the stem cells are the reason; he also exercises religiously and swallows a great many supplements. Research is ongoing. Some predict that a stem cell treatment involving injection of new dopamine-producing cells directly into the brain may be available within five years—to some people, in Europe.

For an off chance, a mere possible, I tell my sister, not far. I'd not sacrifice a great deal. For something proven, not available here but affordable elsewhere,

I'd certainly go above and beyond. But my efforts would not be limitless. I don't want to bankrupt my family. Do I not think I'm worth it? Correct.

If I'm not willing to risk everything for any chance at all, does that mean I am lazy about life? Do I deserve to lose it?

"Would you move to another country?" my sister asks. I can't answer, but I'm very glad to have her to talk with and her questions are to the point. Both of us can be blunt, and neither objects to being on the receiving end of such directness from the other. Our relationship is one that adapts and strengthens in hard times. We grew closer in the maelstrom and aftermath of our parents' decline and deaths, a period when residual resentments, insecurities, and misconceptions were shed. Now, since my diagnosis, we are becoming intimate in new ways. Sometimes it's as if we are telepathic. At this point, I tell her, I'm overwhelmed, and the possible miracle cures feel like a fantasy, and a colossal waste of precious time.

We all have stories about the choices made by the seriously ill. There's a friend who knew she could not bear chemo after the surgery for her cancer and refused it despite her doctors' urgings: still alive and well two decades later. Another woman I knew followed conventional treatment for her disease with what seemed like a world tour of every alternative or emerging option that might possibly help. She tried everything but continued to decline and died within five years. Many of those who loved her spoke of her commitment, bravery, appetite for life. To some, it might seem sad that she spent her last years and months in this way. But that would be from the outside, looking in.

There is a chance that stem cells might come through, or that my "progression" could be like *watching paint dry*. Also possible is that in just a few years I might be far less of my former self or finding so little to enjoy that I'm ready to check out. Or not. I might not care. There is no knowing.

After that first meeting, I don't see Nigel of the red-light hat for many months. When I do, it's in September at an outdoor event in memory of a mutual friend who recently and unexpectedly died. Nigel says all is going well, but I'm shocked by how much worse his tremor and his posture seem, by how quietly he speaks. His facial expression is anxious, haunted; it's a look I remember being shocked by in the mirror when I was at my worst. I worry about his eschewing medical help and then remind myself that of course, this is a sad occasion and, added to that, being in a large group and talking to people one doesn't know well increases stress and so exacerbates symptoms. In any case, all of us have bad days. I remind myself that the disease progresses differently for each of us, that we're all making choices all the time, that Nigel's are, just like mine, the result of what he feels will be best for him and how much he can bear. That he might well be correct about the downside of long-term use of carbidopa/levodopa; that without the flashing helmet and everything else he is doing, his symptoms today might be worse. Again, there is no way of knowing—and no way to quantify the usefulness of *any* of the things we so hopefully do, as citizens of the kingdom of the sick yearning to leave it and return to what used to be our lives.

I've been here, in that other place, for well over a year now. "Welcome," a kindly immigration officer should have said, locking eyes as we, unwilling yet unable to resist, filed up, our miserable grey passports in our shaking hands. "Welcome. Here, you'll learn to accept what you'd love to deny, and to do without many abilities, activities, and certainties you are used to enjoying. Which losses are the most difficult for you, and whether some of them have hidden benefits, will depend on how you think and who you are. Here, this way. Next, please."

4

~

Amplitude

On the screen, Eleanor, slender and immaculate in black and cream sportswear, her dark hair wound into a sleek knot, twists her elegant neck to face her class. My neck (tortoise-like, wrinkled) is already fully cranked so that I can see her, speaker view and full screen, on the laptop propped on my sofa. There are twenty-five of us situated in a variety of living rooms, bedrooms, and basements (most of these rooms seem to be grey or beige), all of us on the floor—actually, floors—and all of us on all fours—no, *threes*, since now our right arms are flung out and up as far as possible, fingers stretching to the ceiling. Various muscles in my chest, armpit, and neck fiercely protest.

"Fling open and up! Let your gaze follow the hand." Eleanor's flawless oval face disappears again as she demonstrates, then explains how next we must curl our flung-open-and-up right arms down and reach them under our bodies and, keeping them parallel to the floor, reach to the left as far as they will go—every fibre and finger should be reaching, she tells us—and then return to all fours. "Open!" she calls, and we collectively yet alone in our rooms, battling our stubborn flesh, unfurl our right arms and again fling them out and up. "Open! Reach! Open! Reach!"

Eleanor is very flexible. Not so the rest of us. We tend to extremes of stiffness and rigidity, also to tremors, depression, and a variety of odd ways of walking. We're taking this class because it's the only thing that might help to slow down the ongoing die-off of cells in our brains that are vital to effective movement, among other things. *Exercise, exercise, and more exercise!* chorus the neurologists, geriatricians, physiatrists, physiotherapists, and all. And not just any exercise. High intensity. Amplitude. Push yourself!

Eleanor recommends forty-five continuous minutes at a minimum of 80 percent of maximum heart rate at least three times a week. Six or seven times is the goal. There should be variety. We need to include movements like these, specifically designed to counteract our muscular-skeletal and neurological symptoms. So here we all are, alone on our floors, collectively reaching and opening in the cause of self-preservation.

"Follow your hand with your gaze!"

As for the 80 percent, an app will monitor your heart rate, but a rule of thumb is that in the 80 percent plus of maximum heart rate zone, a person can speak but will not want protracted conversation. At 95, you're down to monosyllabic grunts and dying on your feet.

"Keep those abdominals and glutes engaged!"

I'm not sure I possess either anymore but do find it oddly relaxing to be told what to do.

"Twenty more. Go! Reach! Open! Reach!" Opening to my left, I notice, is much more difficult than the right. My left arm is where the tremors started. That whole side of my body is stiffer, less alive, less obedient to my commands.

I'm going at a fair pace, though not, I'd say, more than 80 percent. I can feel the work of it—the sensations that come with these peculiar, exaggerated movements that never happen in real life. The need to tighten my abdominals in order not to sway from side to side when I reach up or across. The beginnings of soreness—again, worse on the left where range of movement is restricted.

"Well done!" Oh, these delicious crumbs of praise! How we work for them! "Now, still on all fours . . . Shoot your *right* leg forward and plant it next to your right hand. Then, as you raise your torso, fling both arms back and up. Fingers splayed wide . . . Reach. Squeeze the shoulder blades together. Now back down. Return the leg. Shoot *left* leg forward. Raise and open! Squeeze! Down! Right leg forward . . . Raise, open, squeeze!"

There's a weird, warm almost-pain as my chest opens. My splayed fingers tug against the tightness in my palms. Some abandoned cluster of muscle between my shoulder blades twitches back to life.

"Squeeze! Squeeze! Squeeze!"

We must give ourselves over to the movements we make. We must commit, make them with intention and *amplitude*: maximum extent and range of motion, full effort, awareness of every muscle involved. We need to direct the process, move with purpose, using all our capacity. Be big. Be loud. Thud the feet down. Yell! Be the absolute opposite of what the disease contrives.

Celia, a plump, paisley-bloused woman with hair in a messier version of Eleanor's topknot, unmutes to say that her knees hurt. Earlier, she asked, her voice soft, pleading, that since getting down on the floor took her a long time, could she skip this part? "The more you do it, the easier it will be," Eleanor replied then; now she calmly recommends a folded towel beneath the knees.

You can live well with this, but you'll have to work very hard, wrote Jeanette, a friend of a friend with whom I corresponded shortly after my diagnosis. She sent a link to a television documentary; all of those interviewed spoke of time spent in the gym, cycling, at classes. Motivation, also affected by dopamine deficiency, is a whole other topic. Some of the more affluent had personal trainers.

A trainer with a compatible style (firm and encouraging, rather than hectoring) would leave the exerciser with just one job to do. But, like most people, I can't afford one, so I must be the boss of me. Create an inner Eleanor! Ask myself, *Which is worse? An hour of panting uphill in an awkward half jog or faster degeneration of the substantia nigra?*

You'll need a lot of self-discipline, Jeanette wrote.

Non-writers often tell me how much they admire the "self-discipline" they assume to be involved in writing. The thing is, I enjoy the writing process, and if anything, it's a compulsive activity for me. I'm guessing that those who make this observation experience writing as tedious, or some kind of ordeal: the writer must painfully squeeze words from their heart and brain through their fingers, into the machine and onto the page—and then, after all that effort, the stupid things are not quite what was intended and in the wrong damn order. And then on top of all that, punctuation! Perhaps they imagine it to be like forty-five minutes at 80-plus percent?

Willpower has not, for me, played a large part in writing. Commitment, yes. You learn to turn up at the desk. You learn to be kind to yourself about apparent failures, open to surprises. There's plenty of hard labour and exhaustion, but also a great deal of play involved. The inevitable bad patches are eclipsed by the excitement and pleasure of working with words—I'd say that even now, even at this new slow and uncertain pace. One word leads to the next. Sometimes, to bliss.

But despite me knowing that it is my best chance, that is not yet so with intense (some call it "forced") exercise. At the intensity and duration Eleanor recommends, that 80 percent or more for at least forty-five minutes, you are *continuously* on the edge of wanting, in the moment, to slow down: your body is often saying, *Fuck this!* Over and over, you must remind that body—using your defective, dopamine-deprived and therefore demotivated brain—of the logic behind the enterprise: *Come on! Only another half-hour. Don't complain, it only makes it worse! One minute at a time. It's not so bad at all! It's just new and different. Remember now, we're doing this to stave off ending up in a wheelchair, drooling, demented, and unable to speak or swallow! Remember, there's nothing wrong with being out of breath. But it's okay to back off for half a minute if it lets you keep going. We can do this! We're halfway!*

Et cetera, et cetera, et cetera.

Resistance comes from the body itself. One recent study shows that each jogger or runner has a preferred pace, a speed at which they naturally and comfortably run whatever the terrain. This is also the most efficient, or *energy optimal*, pace for the individual concerned, and it tends to be around 70 percent of maximum heart rate. This makes sense: why would the body waste resources?

Athletes coach and trick themselves into going way beyond this. It's what they need to do to train, improve, compete, and win. They accept it as a tool, become good at it, even addicted to the process.

Can I make that happen to me?

And how much of a reprieve, how much quality of life, will I gain if I do? Impossible to know.

We are on our backs now. Hard to see the screen.

"Arms by your sides. Left arm reach diagonally up, twist, roll. Hand wide open! Pull it back. Back. Right reach, twist, roll. Hand wide open! Pull it back. Big movements! Full control. Are you feeling it?"

Yes. And I do like it: the urgency, the *amplitude*, the gush of my circulation, even the sheer weirdness of it all. And I like the people. I'm starting to recognize the other participants in the tiny boxes at the top of my screen. Occasionally, at the beginning or end of session, a larger form of someone materializes, pores and all, to deliver news or a joke.

A man with frizzy curls who wears the same professorial kind of glasses that I have, but dark blue instead matte black: I like to think he's some kind of scientist, intellectual, or artist. There's a former provincial government minister. There's Len, a lean man of seventy or so, a keener who beams in from a well-equipped garage gym with his gleaming racing bike propped by the door and a purple yoga mat beneath him. There's a telltale waver in his voice. (The vocal folds, like all our muscles, are affected by the disease.) "Eleanor, is this class moderate or high intensity?"

"It's what you make of it, Len. Don't sacrifice your form. Perfect, then build."

Roy, a solid bearded type, exercises in a slate-grey room devoid of any furniture or ornamentation and is sometimes accompanied by his dog. On a different Zoom meeting, "Coping with Your Diagnosis," he described himself as feeling a great reluctance to tackle any of the activities of daily life, something amounting to an *aversion*. I understood his desire to find the best word, felt some kinship with him, and worried when the presenter failed to acknowledge the depth of desperation his vocabulary suggested.

PWP sometimes share a bitter joke to the effect that we rarely end our own lives, due to a chronic lack of drive and motivation. Studies suggest that while thinking about suicide is common in PWP (30 percent), the frequency of suicide in PWP (which, like the general rate, varies a great deal from country to country) is not greater than that of the control populations. In any case, I'm glad that Roy is here now, alive and on the move, along with Helena, a tiny woman who works out, fully and delicately made-up, in her pinkish-grey bedroom; Jacinda and her enormous glossy houseplants; Dave, a very large man whose tiny, trim wife joins him to help with his motivation; and Aso, a hollow-eyed, wispy-haired man with a Buddhist shrine on his sideboard. Not to forget Eleanor herself: lithe and serene, kind, but also stern. How very tidy her kitchen looks.

Naturally, I'd rather be without the disease that has brought me to the floor. On all fours. Standing, seated, prone, and supine; uphill, in water, on bike, outdoors, indoors, online. Yet there are discoveries to be made, people to think about. Fellow exercisers, doctors, instructors, friends of friends of friends.

Eleanor's voice softens as she explains how our disease tightens and stiffens our musculature, making post-workout stretches especially important. We reach above our heads, bend slowly to one side, then the other. We put one foot forward, push the tailbone back, and don't allow our backs to hump. Lift the front foot toes. Interlace our fingers behind our backs as we hinge at the waist. Take a wide stance; shift to the side and feel the lengthening ache the inner thigh. Quadriceps. Hip flexors. Calves. Wrists. Obediently, each muscle targeted responds, and tightness grudgingly becomes relief.

"See you next time! Thank you!" we call out to her and each other until the window whisks away.

I'm not someone who takes pleasure in pain—but I'm also not very elderly. It's true to say that before this hit me, I was more active and fit than most people of my age: hiking, swimming, cycling regularly—for pleasure mainly, but also with a vague notion of keeping fit. It's not that I have *no* willpower. I can to some extent force, coax, or trick myself to do unpleasant things that are good for me. Even so, and despite the strategies I'm taught, I'm finding Eleanor's prescription harder than I expected, particularly when it's just me and the bike or trail. Part of the problem is I suspect that moving at that easier 70 percent that the body prefers is, also for me, a sweet spot for subconscious problem-solving and having ideas, things I very much enjoy.

Well, Eleanor would say, *have you thought that you can do both? Add some 70 percent to your weekly plan!* Routine, she says, is vital.

Mornings, I lace my runners, slip out, and softly close the door. Outside, twice as much light. A scudding sky, a torrent of greens. Pieris, apple, bay, witch hazel, lavender, arbutus, fir, dogwood, currant—leaves beyond number, near, far, in constant motion. I step into a soundscape woven of wind, vegetation, wild bird calls, two roosters, distant engine noise. Inhale: early outsideness, cool and complex, a thrill even to my diseased sense of smell. Oxygen floods in, permeates blood. Squat deep. Rise to standing, arms back, fingers spread, squat, rise, again and again. Heart picks up pace . . .

Don't think, I tell myself. Stay in your body. Just twist, reach, step, jump, stretch, and, of course, breathe. Shrug, roll shoulders loose. Open hands wide. Amplitude. Amplitude.

Crows bicker in the woods. Swallows dive, swoop. A bald eagle wings slowly across, clears the skies for minutes on end. Robin, chickadee, flycatcher, thrush. A scattering of sparrows.

Breathe. Lunge. Count. Twist, reach. Look in the direction of the reach, lift the opposite leg. Contract it all down. Push. Pull. Full on. I start most days this way. And next, as advised by Pauline, a personal trainer friend of a friend, I time a sequence of forty-yard dashes uphill, beginning at 50 percent effort: fast walk, long steps, arms swinging and ending with an all-out sprint. Pauline and I are now in touch every few weeks; it's understood that when I am more settled, in exchange for her training suggestions I'll offer her partner some advice about a novel in progress.

Saunter back. Side stretch, recover. Sixty percent: *very* fast walk, reach with the hips, feet skim the ground. Down, back stretch, recover. Seventy: easy run. Eighty: brisk run. *Look at those weeds there! Going to seed! I could just*—Focus! Ninety: almost full on. Fast, long, sustained. Go! Not bad. Full on, now! Long, fast. More! The leaves blur. 8.2 seconds. Good. Suck in the morning air, and set out the tape to measure for some long jumps.

"Work out for your life!" Pauline instructs. "Focus on developing *raw power!*" She instinctively distrusts and disapproves of all medication but concedes that I, not she, live in/with this body and brain.

To make a hike deliver *high intensity*, I must stride vigorously up a mountain trail, taking no rests for a continuous forty-five minutes, and jog where the gradient is not steep enough. It's a heart-pumping, gasping kind of thing, but the richness of the environment really helps; even so, not everyone enjoys hiking with me. My artist friend and I are compatible, but when joined by her less active friend, we hit a barrier minutes in.

"I'll call this a day," she gasps. "You two go on!" We don't, of course; we negotiate a slower pace and a shorter route to an enticing lookout. There's time to look around. We watch siskins skitter from tree to tree, notice a clutch of late oyster mushrooms growing in layers from the rotting trunks of fallen alder. We stop to watch a ceanothus silk moth the size of a small hand slowly fan its new wings dry at the side of the trail, a thing none of us have seen before.

There's the soft hiss of a brief shower so we stop again to listen to it falling without the distraction of our footsteps, then continue through fern and glistening thigh-high salal, a steep cliff to our left. There's time and breath to talk about our daughters, about recent local conflicts between neighbours over some crowing roosters, the absurdity of local building regulations. We veer from the terrifying climate crisis to the stupidity of all levels of government—a phenomenon so outrageous that, to avoid the opposite, we must laugh.

Our shoulders loose, our skin just faintly damp, we settle on the rocky knoll with the baby Garry oak tree that's picked an awful spot and is doomed to be a bonsai. The valley spreads beneath us, and beyond it the sea, other islands, the horizon. A single cloudlet in the sky. Oh, yes, there must be this too. Pleasure, wonder, companionship. Gossip. A different kind of amplitude.

"Yes, of course," Eleanor says. "Make sure to also leave time for it."

When it's impractical to be outside, I climb awkwardly onto the ancient stationary bike we bought fifth-hand and hauled up into what used to be my husband's workshop—now "the gym." The bike was designed for giants: height adjusts well enough, but the distance from the excruciating seat to handlebars is a stretch and as well as that the mechanism whirs and whines once you start.

I shove a bit of foam between bony butt and hard seat, play Tanya Tagaq's "Uja," Fela Kuti's "Zombie" and "Roforofo Fight." I need my heart to accelerate, lungs to fill right up; I need my blood to absorb the O_2, quit dawdling and do the chemistry, rush fuel to the cells that crave it, learn to enjoy discomfort because of what it will bring to me. The heart is not particularly keen. There's a familiar mummified feeling in my thighs. I'm stuck in the low-70 percentages and feel like total shit for minutes on end.

But the display will and does hit the 80 mark, 85. I push it: 90, 95, back down to 85. Haul the breath in, gasp it out. Warm, then hot. Toss the jacket. Sweat beads my chest. My heart wants out. *Stop this!* meat-me cries out. But no. 80. 85.

Outside, just a boring patch of scrappy trees, driveway, and occasional dowdy sparrow. *But at least you have a window!* Window, display, window. There's mental math. There's getting there, then there's almost done . . . And perhaps—just perhaps—I'm feeling a little less resistance, both mental and physical.

Cool-down comes: a crystalline clear-headedness, a mixture of relief and something sweeter still.

I have studied the information Eleanor sent and tunnelled into the internet. The title of Dr. J. Alberts's 2009 landmark study says it all: "Forced, Not Voluntary, Exercise Improves Motor Function in Parkinson's Disease Patients." The powerful and even neurogenerative effects of exercise at a "forced" or high-intensity pace is proven, as is its considerable benefit to people with a variety of neurological disorders. All doctors recommend it. I remember again the neurologist, how he smiled and leaned forward as he recommended "exercise, exercise, and more exercise."

So push the creaking pedals down, press the up arrows, sweat. A damp breeze wafts through the window, along with scraps of birdsong. Push! Push!

Yet I cannot help thinking, Could all this exercise *also* be a distraction or mere coping mechanism? A kind of denial? A raft to cling to: *At least I'm doing something.*

Yes. I'm sure it is all of these. And why not? Bring it on! Because there is a lot to deal with here and few instructions as to how to square up to the existential and emotional dimensions of this unexpected and unwelcome experience. Practical remedies like exercise and nutrition, even recommendations to focus on the many good things one experiences, to practice mindfulness, meditation, and so on may help; they are not enough.

What confronts me is an extreme form of what we *all* need to cope with as we age and acknowledge our mortality, yet it does differ from that more general expectation of slow decline and eventual death in that it's happening in my relative youth, and noticeably fast. There's a rough-and-ready time scale, a strong likelihood of some undesirable outcomes, and, unfortunately, Parkinson's is not a vaccination against other illnesses or other kinds of misfortune. Indeed, it makes me more vulnerable to other unpleasant medical conditions such as melanoma, heart failure, osteoporosis, orthostatic hypotension, and—goodness, I nearly forgot—dementia. I could *also* be run over by a bus, suffer an aneurysm or heart attack, or develop an aggressive form of cancer—just as many people do every day.

My lurking symptoms are a reminder of the likely shape of things to come; so are the medications taken at intervals throughout the day to suppress them. Some may find full-on denial useful protection when confronted with this blend of unwanted change, new knowledge, and uncertainty as to which kind of bad thing will happen next, but I don't think that will work for me any more than will chasing hypothetical remedies.

So how to live with the prospect of losses ahead? How best to proceed without any real sense of how quickly or with what sets and sequences of symptoms this degenerative process will unfold for me, though I know the horrifying range of possibilities and the inevitability of the general direction—that is, worse? Apart from *keep moving*, which does take a considerable part of every day, what will I do with whatever amount of fairly good time I have?

These are not easy questions and I suspect no response will be final.

I know that I need to observe and explore. Learn. Put that despicable passport to good use.

And yes, *keep moving*.

5

~

Trouble with Words

I've been on medication for six months when Alex and I run into each other on the path to the high school gymnasium–cum–voting station. I'm on my way out, she's going in. Our children who used to play together are now adults, and because of the pandemic, it's been ages since Alex and I have even glimpsed each other off-screen. She's been sick too. Her face is thinner; her new hair thicker and darker.

"I've been given the all-clear," she says. "Next checkup in six months, then every year. Let me tell you, this has been such a journey." It seems to me that Alex gives the word *journey* a special resonance, a kind of audible halo, and after saying it, she pauses, maintaining eye contact longer than I find comfortable. It's as if the word is coded or magical in some way. *Journey.* Trapped in her gaze, I feel a prickly rush of panic and irritation at her use of this word, try to cast it aside. *Ease up*, I instruct myself. It's her experience; she'll describe it as she wants. We're engaged in conversation, not literary criticism or a vocabulary test. It's just a word. *Journey.*

My quarrel is not with Alex, and not even with the word, but with the many people who now use it to describe almost any difficult or even mildly effortful process of change: a disease, a degree, a divorce, weight loss.

One might ask, Doesn't *journey* connect rather well with the notion of sickness as involuntary exile, another country, travel, distance from home, new language, new undesirable passport, that cluster of imagery I've been so enamoured with? Somewhat. But it's baggy, vague, unspecific—

As these thoughts churn inchoately inside me, I hear Alex say that she has returned to work and is loving it; everyone at the bank has been totally supportive. That she is running again. How as soon as it's possible to travel again, she and Mark will splash out on a truly extravagant holiday. She's not sure, but perhaps the Caribbean? Or what about Costa Rica: it has green values but also, now, some more luxurious yet also sustainable options—

"Wonderful!" I gush. "Great news! And you do look so well!"

I'm utterly sincere, but even as the words emerge, they feel extraordinarily clichéd: two stock phrases stapled together *and* a typical, cringe-inducing feminine way to connect—over appearance. So banal!

Yet Alex's smile makes it very clear that I've said the right thing. I would say her smile is infectious, but I've backed myself into a tight corner cliché-wise. It touches every part of her face, and me too. We pass it back and forth between us, make warm, preverbal happy sounds in our throats, then via a few minor observations and questions, switch to an exchange of news.

It strikes me now, remembering this conversation with Alex, how much my relationship to language, both written and spoken, has changed since I was diagnosed. I approach new vocabulary with more caution, less delight. It's another loss. Or should I, as sick people are supposed to do, reframe that more positively as a *challenge* or even a *learning opportunity*?

The disease itself, although far from providing a verbal treasure trove, has the rudiments of some informal usage of its own. They are hardly inventive or exciting, but I do appreciate the lack of pretension. For example, *on* or *on-times* for when medication is working and symptoms are under control, and *off*, naturally, for the opposite. (My friend Linda uses *locked out*, better, I think, because it adds feeling.) Short, simple, and practical.

I'm fine, too, with *Sinemet honeymoon*, which old-timers use for the years at the beginning of their treatment (the years I am living now) when a now-discontinued brand of the most common medication, carbidopa/levodopa, consistently worked.

As with any physical malfunction, there's a torrent of nasty medical jargon referring to symptoms—*festination* (having to walk very fast), *hypomimia* (loss of facial expressiveness), *dystonia* (cramps and spasms), *sialorrhea* (drooling), *akathisia* (a strange, almost electrical, almost burning, utterly maddening feeling known as restless leg syndrome), *bradykinesia* (slowness of all movements), *dyskinesia* (erratic writhing involuntary movements), *micrographia* (that shrinking and weakening of one's handwriting), and so on, ad nauseam. There are even, I'm shaken to discover, some Parkinson's symptoms that present via spoken and written word use. The rather jolly-sounding *verbigeration* refers to the compulsive repetition of seemingly meaningless words, phrases, or sentences.

Logorrhea, a communication disorder that causes excessive "wordiness" and repetition in speech, sometimes to the point of incoherence, can be a side effect of certain Parkinson's medications. It's used more casually to mean over-elaborate speech in general, what used to be called *prolixity*.

Graphorrhea is a similar disorder occurring specifically in written work. It is associated with schizophrenia but can also result from other psychiatric and neurological disorders (*not* Parkinson's so far as I'm aware). Graphorrheaic written ramblings may follow some or all grammatical rules yet still leave the reader confused as to what the piece is about: a writer's nightmare!

Almost any word except *euphoria* that ends with "ia" or "ea" is bad news.

Various parts of the brain have lovely, mysterious-sounding names, but their meanings turn out to be less gorgeous than their sound. For example, the substantia nigra—the origin of most of the tiny quantity of dopamine-creating neurons in the brain—and the associated nigrostriatal pathway initially intrigued me. But *substantia nigra* translates from Latin as "the black stuff." (Oddly enough, this was the title of a 1980s TV drama about men who lay asphalt that I remember watching.) It turns out that because dopamine-producing cells are associated with a high concentration of neuromelanin, this small region of the brain is indeed naturally blackish (the rest is pinkish grey). Utterly fascinating! But wait! I have also to take on that *my* dopamine-producing cells in *my* substantia nigra are disintegrating . . .

Likewise, I'm less than thrilled to learn that the cuddly-sounding *Lewy bodies* are abnormal deposits of the protein alpha-synuclein; they negatively affect both movement and mood and cause cognitive impairment, hallucinations, delusions—a kind of dementia that has about a 50 percent chance of afflicting me in the long term, depending, perhaps, on how long the long term is.

It's best to pace encounters with this kind of information, but I don't like feeling so cautious. It's not how I used to be. It reminds me there is something wrong with me, and of William Blake's poem "The Sick Rose."

> *O Rose thou art sick.*
> *The invisible worm,*
> *That flies in the night*
> *In the howling storm:*
>
> *Has found out thy bed*
> *Of crimson joy:*
> *And his dark secret love*
> *Does thy life destroy.*

So yes, I'm having trouble with words. And whatever a journey is, it is *not* a trip or tour. A journeyer is likely travelling a long way into territory previously unknown. The journey will involve effort, risk, self-reliance, uncertainty, a confrontation with difficult or outright dangerous circumstances. The destination may be a place aspired to or unknown.

A journey can be a self-chosen adventure full of discovery, learning, pleasure; it may be perilous and traumatic. Often it's a blend of both.

When refugees, migrants, or asylum seekers set out on foot, in trucks and lorries, in overloaded boats with fake or inadequate or no life jackets, only to arrive in a new place where more suffering awaits, they are indeed making a journey, but the word in this instance and given current usage now seems wrong. More appropriately, *escape. Flight. Ordeal.*

There is a long history of arduous travel in search of healing. Pilgrimages to holy places are still made, as they were traditionally, on foot by the sick and by believers of various kinds. Some pilgrims walk on bare feet or even on their knees, for at least the last part of the route. Suffering is part of pilgrimage, though if the sick pilgrim cannot walk, then they may be carried. The current (mis)use of *journey* taps into this tradition.

British author Raynor Winn's first memoir, *The Salt Path,* charts a six-hundred-mile coastal hike through Somerset, Devon, and Cornwall in England. Winn and her husband, Moth, committed to it in response to the triple disaster that wiped out their former lives: bankruptcy, the loss of their home, and his diagnosis of corticobasal degeneration, a horrible and rapidly "progressive" neurological disorder sometimes known as "Parkinson's plus."

They have almost no money, so skimp on food and camp wild. Winn viscerally evokes the land- and seascapes, along with the physical and psychological effects of constant walking and living outside: daily struggles with fatigue, hunger, and extremes of weather punctuated with more lyrical descriptions of their natural surroundings. She details their encounters with human and animal others, and charts the profound ways in which they are changed by the experience—including unexpected improvements in her husband's symptoms.

Theirs was a journey at the same time literal and figurative. However, it's striking that although *journey* appears on the jacket copy of the book, it's not a word Winn uses much, if at all. Others they encounter use the symbolically laden "the path," which forms part of the book's title. Winn and Moth mainly think and speak of what they are doing as "the walk." The narrative focuses on the physical, practical aspects and emotional impact of doing what they have agreed to undertake and wisely leaves it to the reader to add italics or a spiritual gloss, or not.

A journey may be undertaken for many reasons—in the spirit of adventure; as a quest; perhaps in the hope of finding a particular plant, person, form of knowledge, lost object; or even in the pursuit of pleasure—but the seriously ill are not in the main voluntary travellers. Winn and Moth choose to walk because nothing of their old life remains to hold them in place.

When *journey* is used in the context of serious illness, it's not necessarily a reference to actual travels. It is instead, or at the same time, a metaphor for a protracted experience of suffering, learning, and changing: for how much, during sickness and treatment, you undergo. For the distance between what you once were and what you become as your disease and your attempts to deal with it continue. It suggests how very different (far away) you are at the end (death) from your former self and former condition (ease, aliveness).

Journey gained verbal currency in the context of cancer as a less combative alternative to *fight, beat, battle with.* And it has now become the norm to talk of any long-lasting, serious, and especially terminal illness as if it took place on horseback or on board a catamaran. The *Parkinson's* journey: here we go, shuffling, tripping, stumbling, and festinating down the path . . .

~

I do see that the illness-as-journey trope makes an appropriate connection between the danger, suffering, difficulty, and uncertainty met on the trail with the tortuous malfunctions which can afflict a body. And the metaphor of illness as journey may be comforting in its open-endedness: on such an expedition, anything is possible, even a cure, a miracle. *Journey* suggests that on the involuntary way from disease to cure or horrible early death, there will be agonies and losses—but also, perhaps, the possibility of growth, of compensatory spiritual gains. Redemption even. That suffering will be good for you, even in some way *worth it.*

It's here that, for me, this characterization of disease slips beyond metaphor—beyond overwrought cliché—into cringe-worthy euphemism: it minimizes suffering, reeks of cover-up, and, worse still, it aims to guide the sufferer as to what to make of their experience, to suggest that they will—or should—find the spiritual silver lining, part of which might be to eventually feel grateful for something that at first sight has nothing to recommend it.

Now this may be a sensible, even inevitable adjustment to circumstances. I may do so. May even have begun to. I don't dismiss Eve Joseph's view that while euphemism, associated with denial, "helps us to avoid forbidden topics, it also offers a way to voice the unspeakable." However, in this case, the pretense and cover-up outrage me, in the same way that the fluffy pink bunnies of aggressive "positive thinking" infuriated the late Barbara Ehrenreich. Must we constantly be exhorted to apply a positive gloss on everything, even agony and devastating losses?

Turn up the cooling, please . . .

I feel better for having written this down.

~

We seek out metaphor because our individual experience can be very difficult to convey to another person. Confronted by something that feels new and significant, we reach for comparison, for an image, some other thing or action that's in some way similar, a like-ness that might help a listener or reader, and even the writer, to *see,* as we put it, what we are hoping to convey.

Linguist Elena Semino at Lancaster University in the UK has studied the way people with cancer use metaphor, and notes that when we choose a metaphor, we take a particular perspective on what is described. "In the 'battle' metaphor for cancer, the disease is an enemy; in the 'journey' metaphor, it is usually the road we travel on." When talking about life-threatening disease, Semino points out, the same metaphor can be a source of understanding and empowerment, or the reverse.

I should note that for me the "road we travel on" is also euphemistic and squirm-inducing, whereas "enemy" merely seems prosaic and inadequate.

"Cancer is like an unexpected lodger," noted a participant in one of Semino's workshops. One who "messes everything up, and causes chaos. Then just when you finally get rid of them and close the door, you realize they've kept the key." A similar image drives Shaena Lambert's brilliant and avowedly autobiographical story "Oh, My Darling," written in the aftermath of her cancer treatment. It features the voice of an uninvited guest who inhabits the main character: a voice constantly, hypnotically announcing the suffering to come and the inevitability of her surrender. Writing this story, the author told me, was an intense and compelling experience. Unwelcome, overwhelming, and even horribly seductive as that voice was, writing the story offered her an opportunity to distance her now-recovered self from her illness—to feel not mastery but a level-headed sense of empowerment because she had thus far been able to resist and was equal to a major threat to her existence, and could use it as material.

Semino's study focused on cancer, but the "uninvited guest" metaphor is accommodating and versatile. It can be customized to fit almost any serious illness, including Parkinson's. François Gravel's brisk and bossy but far from evil Colonel Parkinson, as characterized in his memoir *Colonel Parkinson in Charge*, seems relatively benign and may have helped his creator retain his good humour and equanimity following his diagnosis. Peter Dunlap-Shohl's personification of the disease in "Interview with a Killer," the third chapter of his graphic novel *My Degeneration*, takes the form of a green-skinned bureaucrat in a suit and tie.

"What do you want from me?" the Dunlap-Shohl character asks.

"Everything it has taken you a lifetime to acquire, learn," the increasingly ominous bureaucrat calmly replies, before launching into a relentless, heart- and gut-wrenching list and concluding, "I want it all, your entire self, the physical and emotional. . . . I am the thug who is going to kick your pathetic ass and leave it for the crows!"

I imagine Dunlap-Shohl felt at the end of this scene the wonderful rush of catharsis: that intense and physical release that follows when we express without restraint and concern for others the full awfulness of our situation and how horrible it feels.

I don't so far have an image of an uninvited guest. If I did, I might think of her as both beastly and human: a hybrid creature, part human, part she-wolf, not yet mature. Sometimes she seems more human; at others, more animal. Secretive, solitary, always hungry. Sharp face, small features. Sly eyes. Parts of her body thatched with wiry hair, or even unkempt feathers—there's a dry rustling that could be feathers or her breath. She neither speaks nor howls. If she had not long ago stolen my ability to smell, I might notice a faint, woody musk: the scent detectable only by human super-smellers, and dogs, of Parkinson's. A bitter beast. Speechless, cunning. Secretive. Driven to destroy, even if that means she, too, will die. Unless when done with me, she materializes in someone else.

I have no scruples about the uninvited guest. It's easy and in a way satisfying to flesh out a personification like this. But for me it's only an experiment. I don't want to continue. I don't feel that casting my disease as a monster will help me. It might even be counterproductive, a waste of dwindling imaginative resources, to give the disease more life and space than it has already stolen.

Stolen? A thief, then? Perhaps the kind of thief who, in broad daylight and equipped only with a few multi-purpose tools, silently and swiftly removes the pane of glass from your window, squeezes through without leaving a mark, replaces the glass, then, gloved, examines every cranny and nook deciding what to take— No. I'm not feeling it.

Do I lack skill with absolute villains because the former novelist in me wants to award them a sympathetic streak, a soupçon of vulnerability, some humanizing charm or quirk—wants to create sympathy for the devil who represents the disease? Whereas the rest of me, living the reality rather than inhabiting the metaphor, cannot conceive of doing so? Or maybe, since things—since *I*—keep changing, I don't yet grasp the scale of what I'm up against and it's too early for the experience to crystallize into an analogy? Or is this, like the novel writer's extended use of imagination, something I think I don't *want* to do but actually *can't*? Am I losing another writerly skill?

This is not a pleasant thought, but I'm hoping my undiminished ability to judge and criticize others militates against it. Even the passport, exile to another country—all of that sometimes seems less compelling. How come the new country has so much of the old one in it? What degree of wellness qualifies one for a return home? What kind of passports do our families have? The more I ponder it, the more it needs to be clarified.

There is however another side to all this. For all that I loathe it, that grey passport has brought me to encounters with the writings of other inhabitants and their physicians whose words have exhilarated and touched me, added dimension and perspective to my experience. I'm thinking not just of classics of the genre—the work of Virginia Woolf, Oliver Sacks, Susan Sontag, Joan Didion—but also of contemporary writers like Hilary Mantel who wrote novel after novel despite acute pain from endometriosis, pausing only when hospitalized to condense her experience of decades of torturous pain, medical mismanagement, and what she learned from it into the fifteen-page essay "Meeting the Devil."

"Illness strips you back to an authentic self, but not one you need to meet," she warns.

Writers' perspectives on sickness naturally differ widely according to their character and the nature of their malady. Virginia Woolf writes elegantly in *On Being Ill* of the inadequacy of language to convey pain. The sufferer, she says, "is forced to coin words himself, and, taking his pain in one hand, and a lump of pure sound in the other . . . so to crush them together that a brand new word in the end drops out." Reading this, I was somewhat skeptical, even as I appreciated her well-crafted metaphor. I merely noted that few women speak in whole sentences as labour progresses and perhaps pure sound could be a very eloquent response to pain? Mantel, however, is outraged:

> I can't understand what [Woolf] means when she complains about the "poverty of the language" we have to describe illness. . . . What

of the whole vocabulary of stinging aches, of spasms, of strictures and cramps; the gouging pain, the drilling pain, the pricking and pinching, the throbbing, burning, stinging, smarting, flaying? . . . No one's pain is so special that the devil's dictionary of anguish has not anticipated it.

Confronted by a request to rate her pain on a scale of one to ten, Eula Biss answers with a twenty-page explanation of how this is impossible. "The pain scale measures only the intensity of pain, not the duration," she writes. "This may be its greatest flaw. A measure of pain, I believe, requires at least two dimensions. The suffering of Hell is terrifying not because of any specific torture, but because it is eternal."

There's disagreement, but also co-creation: Woolf's "undiscovered countries" of sickness become in Susan Sontag's hands that "other place," the kingdom of the sick, to which she contributes the passport. When Rebecca Solnit encounters the idea, she further elaborates and deepens the image. "In this country," she writes, "you are yourself the terrain, and you are travelling toward or away from your own mortality . . . House, country, landscape, kingdom of the body, now strange and foreign."

Even as she used and played with metaphor, Sontag famously warned against using diseases as metaphors: speaking of one thing in terms of another is intended to illuminate, but it may instead spread dangerous misunderstanding.

Writer and editor Anatole Broyard, not a man to restrain himself, wrote with characteristic bravado in response to his cancer diagnosis that being sick was comparable to "a visit to a disturbed country, rather like contemporary China." He also conceived of it as "a love affair with a demented woman who demanded things I had never done before." "Metaphors," he continued, "may be as necessary to illness as they are to literature, as comforting to the patient as his own bathrobe and slippers. At the very least, they are a relief from medical terminology."

I enjoy the slippers and hope Broyard did, though he did not return from his visit to the other country. Eve Joseph's memoir takes us to what lies beyond it: death. She acknowledges Sontag's position on metaphor but adds, "the use of metaphor . . . makes room for the imagination. It allows the mind to walk toward death without having to confront it directly."

The perfect aptness of a metaphor is not the only good that may emerge from a writer's attempt to stretch language. If I part company with some aspect of the connection between image and actuality, that, too, may be interesting and enrich the read. Faced with the task of conveying raw experience, we're driven to poetry, analogy; we tap into existing metaphors, elaborate them, invent new ones. Make fresh combinations of words, try out new usages, reject them, resort to pure sound. Try, fail, try again. Some will do whatever it takes to communicate, to offer something, some meaning, to push back against isolation.

I'd be bereft without the work of the writers who have shown me how alteration, suffering, and loss can be endured, described, mined for meaning, made into something beautiful (often funny, too), then shared as part of an ongoing written conversation. Their words have sustained me with a blend of aesthetic pleasure and factual or emotional learning and, even more important, the miraculous feeling of communication and connection. Reading, I'm joined not only to the writer but also to others who have and will read the same words. My solitary experience is validated, dignified, acknowledged as part of a complicated human whole. I'd go so far as to say that this kind of writing and reading experience is a kind of love, vital in its own way, though of course it does not offer the intimacy and lived history of exchanges with family and friends.

"Both of us were fortunate in our bodies—felt our bodies were indeed ourselves," writes one dear friend, now in her eighties, her mobility and eyesight deserting and limiting her even as her full faculties remain. "We experienced a great deal of pleasure (and, no doubt, pride) in their beauty and perfect functioning. It's a shock when this ends. I now think of my body as 'brother ass': something I force, something I feel pity for, something I wonder how far I should push.

I'm no longer the self I was—but something survives and struggles on. Tries to enjoy what there is to appreciate, and succeeds most, if not all, of the time."

Sickness can be a compelling subject. Writing on the topic spans a broad spectrum from astonishing and uplifting via a useful-but-not-exciting middle ground of textbooks and information sharing and on to what one of my editors calls *dreck*: vapid and infuriating. The middle ground is where much of the unpleasant vocabulary I need to absorb is explained in tomes like *The New Parkinson's Disease Treatment Book: Partnering with Your Doctor to Get the Most from Your Medications*. As this title suggests, these books are detailed, thorough, worthy, and dense. In a word, *heavy*. Avoid overload. Reading is a mission. Go in. Extract what's useful. Mark page. Exit.

After this comes a rapid descent: well-intended articles, columns, and newsletters focused on ways to cope, self-help, and attempted humour that dissolve into a quagmire of imprecision, vogue phrases, and relentless cliché. *My journey. Your journey. Her journey.* It's everywhere: news, friends, the internet, even *doctors*! That I must struggle so hard to justify the frustration it engenders in me makes it even worse.

~

Alex and I, still standing on the brick path beside the gymnasium, feel a sudden chill as the sun begins to drop below the treeline. It's time to wind up our exchange.

"So good to catch up and hear your great news," I say. "And I hope you get that holiday soon!"

She touches me on the shoulder. "Thank you. Good luck with *your* journey, Kathy," she says, her voice soft, sympathetic. And I know! I absolutely do know she's offering kinship, goodwill, encouragement. And I'm grateful. Or know that I ought to be. But this is now *my* experience we are talking about. *Journey? We're not on a [expletive] sailing trip!*

I thank Alex and hurry to the car. I refrain from yelling or banging my fist on the steering wheel, instead ask myself, *What is this? Why can't I let it go? Am I jealous of her remission? Of her having a disease that is, just sometimes, cured?* I really don't think so. I'm just mad about words. And no, this is not logorrhea! Tired approximations and threadbare clichés actually have the opposite effect to that intended by the speaker or writer. They muffle what is being said. They fray the connection that we hope to create when considering something vital to us both. They protect us from thinking and feeling. And they make me want to scream.

A life spent writing, reading, and listening has spoiled me not only for the uninvited guest and for the *journey* but also for many other apt yet overused expressions. Yet despite the intensity of my feelings here, I do acknowledge that literature and life, mutually dependent, are not the same thing. I remind myself that in moments of extremity or intense emotion, or when homes are destroyed and survivors tell their stories, it is mainly stock phrases that emerge. *A wall of flames. A raging inferno. My heart sank. The sun was blotted out. One minute everything was fine, the next— Time stood still. It was like the end of the world.*

In times of great loss, meaning flows back into apt but outworn expressions and they seem true again. So it's possible, even likely, that as my difficulties become more acute, I will find that plain, ordinary words; roughly fitting, well-used phrases; and even squirm-inducing metaphors are good enough— perhaps at times better—than nuanced and original phrasings that draw attention to themselves. After all, sweating, terrified, I'm unlikely to waste my time gazing at the approaching forest fire while I struggle for alternatives to "wall of flames" or choose an original way to convey the ghastly, devouring sound it makes. Since I want to communicate, somehow, anyhow, whatever it takes, I may perhaps be glad of whatever first comes to mind.

Perhaps. Maybe. Meanwhile, I have good reasons for being very passionate about words, and I am not on any kind of journey.

Others have every right to feel differently. And to use that word.

I offer both thanks and apologies to Alex, who, on a sunny September afternoon, feeling happy and meaning only the best, unknowingly became the target of my frustration and rage—about the use of words but also, I suspect, about having a horrible disease.

I appreciate her good wishes, and I'm glad that she unwittingly prompted me to begin to think about the *J*-word. I hope her good news becomes better still. I wish her a hammock in the shade of a guanacaste tree, mornings of wild birdsong, and, on the last rainforest day, a longed-for sighting of the very rare quetzal. And of course, a yellow-sand beach and warm nights listening to the ocean's gentle breath.

Ssh, aah, ssh, aah, ssh aah . . .

6

~

The Exquisite Cyclops

Another telehealth appointment, six months after diagnosis. We're deep into Covid times. Not fun at all, but on we go. I'm at the kitchen table, phone on speaker, notepad and pen to hand. The doctor has a quiet, rather sad voice.

"Do you have vivid dreams?"

"No," I say. "The thing is, I hardly sleep. I'm exhausted. Is there anything—"

"But you do!" Richard shouts from the new home office.

I'd assumed he was out, so I'm doubly startled when he appears atop the short flight of stairs leading to the kitchen.

"You really do—every night. You talk, mutter, yell. Thrash around." He runs his fingers through his hair. *Sorry*, he mouths at me.

I turn back to the phone. "So apparently I do."

The doctor sighs. "Well, we're normally paralyzed during REM sleep and that prevents us from acting out our dreams. But quite often, with this condition—"

Condition? I think. It's not a pregnancy! What century are we in?

"—your REM sleep is disordered, so paralysis doesn't always occur. You act out your dreams. These dreams tend to be aggressive and can be dangerous. Are you injuring yourself or anyone else?"

I glance back over my shoulder. Richard has vanished. "Not so far as I know."

There are treatments, apparently, but they're quite problematic. The doctor advises me to stay on the same dose of medication for now. "Let's add this to the watch list: rapid eye movement sleep behaviour disorder."

I find Richard outside, stacking firewood.

"But why didn't you tell me?"

"I don't know. I forget, and then I don't want to bother you with it . . . And sometimes, yes, you're sort of running or struggling, even yelling, but most of the time, you're just muttering away to yourself. Now and then you scream."

"Scream?"

"Or laugh. Sometimes I can make out a sentence."

So even though *I* am oblivious to them, my dreams are waking *him*!

Not really, he says. Only briefly. Doesn't bother him. "The cat is far more of a problem." He smothers a yawn.

I offer to sleep in the spare room, and I mean it, but I'm relieved when he says, quite vehemently, *no.*

I would miss him dreadfully. When I'm awake, I can tell if he is alert too. Sleeping, he lies on his left side, and if there's any light, I am reassured by the shape he makes next to me, head to shoulder, waist to toe.

Some writers and artists claim to have been inspired by dreams, but my dream recall has always been sparse. Periodically I discover an extra room in my house (a different one each time); occasionally I recall more complex scenarios.

As a fiction writer, I had excellent daytime access to my subconscious, something I retained from child-hood, when it was encouraged, and developed through constant use. Symbols, questions, storylines, dialogue, interaction between invented characters—all that popped up while I was fully conscious. Because I spent a lot of my waking hours imagining things, some of them very bizarre—waking dreams, effectively—I thought that perhaps I did not need access to the sleep-ing kind?

Since I became ill, I haven't been able to work imaginatively. It's enough of a challenge describing what's right in front of me. But I miss the invented characters, locations, events—especially the surreal and extraordinary. The alleged drama of my current sleep-scape, the sheer energy of it all, makes me very curious. It's infuriating to be providing so much entertainment and yet be excluded from the party.

I could record my nocturnal shouts and mutterings with my phone. Instead, I select a notebook with a wavy design on the cover and good hand feel, one that opens easily; I add a new soft pencil and arrange this equipment on my nightstand as an invitation. I remind myself nightly to pay attention.

Every morning, I wake exhausted, remember pre-cisely nothing, and later ask my husband for his report.

"*'How dare you!'* I think that was it."

"Humming. You sounded happy."

"You said, 'Would you like one of these?'"

These what? Miniature falafel? Olives? Prawns? Heated face cloth held out with tongs?

"A loud scream."

"You yelled, 'You bastard! You've always been like this!' I hope it wasn't me."

I remember none of it. Would it help to *invent* some dreams incorporating these fragments of dia-logue? Maybe. But what I yearn for is an actual dream, in colour, with weird people, flowers, extraterrestrial visitors, sex . . .

"Muttering—then you said in a bored voice, 'Et cetera, et cetera, et cetera.'"

"You said we would be late."

Bus, train, or plane? Transatlantic liner? Been there, done that, dream. Yawn.

"You said no thanks, it really wasn't your thing."

Bondage? Country music? Fermented seal meat?

"Making some complicated arrangements."

"You asked, 'Do you want to join us?'"

In the swimming pool? In bed? A voyage to Argentina?

"You spoke very clearly and confidently in a foreign language. Finnish?"

"You laughed! A deep chuckle. Said, 'Come on, now!'"

This sounds better, but of course I remember *nothing*—even when I scream myself awake, and our adult son rushes to our bedroom.

"Are you all right, Mum? What's going on?" None of us know. *Bloodcurdling* is how he describes the scream.

My exhausted husband turns back onto his left side.

"Sorry . . . can't . . . help . . ."

So it goes, until, deeply asleep, I'm visited by a woman endowed with a single eye, large and exquisite, in the middle of her forehead. The iris is a complex composition of blue, brown, and gold; the lid and socket sumptuously curved; the sole eyebrow long and arched. The rest of the face (which I assume to belong to a woman, though that need not be the case) is harmoniously arranged around this central eye and subtly made-up to accentuate its features: a wide mouth with full lips the colour of plums, angled cheekbones, a strong jaw, gleaming golden-brown hair cut to echo it.

Though located exactly mid-forehead, pupil dead centre, the eye's little fleshy nodule containing the tear duct in the left corner renders the face asymmetrical. And yet the overall effect is one of balance. She's strange and beautiful. Mysterious, powerful.

Hers could be the face of a goddess, of an alien queen. An exquisite cyclops. Though can I call her that? Cyclopes are by reputation not only one-eyed but also gigantic, violent, and slow-witted, none of which apply to this woman.

"Who are you?" My voice, loud inside my skull, wakes me, and I lie in thick darkness remembering her over and over and promising to record her in my book. While Richard breathes evenly beside me, I deliberately imagine that he and I are sitting on a green plaid blanket laid out on sun-dappled ground beneath ancient Garry oaks. We're sharing a picnic of berries and other fruit when the exquisite cyclops reappears wearing—like us—a white tunic and wide-legged pants. I invite her to join us. She nods, sits.

"Who are you?" I ask again.

"Who do you want me to be?" Her voice vibrates like a cello.

Awake in the semi-dark of our bedroom, I try to answer. I know I don't want her to be anyone I can identify. I don't care that the internet interprets dreams of a one-eyed person as a sign that I'm not seeing the whole picture, or that I'm being seduced by a demon. I've had a dream! One with no yelling or violence at all! I almost rouse Richard to tell him.

A by-product of rapid eye movement sleep behaviour disorder is (even more) exhaustion, but when Covid-19 restrictions ease and we're invited to a party, I'm keen to go. At least thirty people—an intoxicating experience after months of isolation—spill into the overgrown garden, eating, drinking, catching up. After an hour or so, I'm drawn to someone I haven't met before, Phyllis: a graceful, brightly dressed older woman who has one leg. Her foot emerges from beneath a rustling silk skirt, encased in a fuchsia running shoe. She pats the cushion next to her, and I sit. She hovers her hand an inch or so above my wrist, something I have seen her do to several others. Do I feel anything? She tells me my energy is low and uneven. *Ragged.*

"Energy? What energy?" I say, and suddenly I am explaining my recent diagnosis, the long wait to receive it, and how, between the disease, the recommended exercise regime, and the various sleep interruptions, I don't have a lot left in me.

"I can't cure you," she says, "but maybe I can make things easier. I used to be a nurse. What I do now is therapeutic touch." She suggests I look it up online and get back to her if interested.

Touch that is not actually touch. It's not something I would naturally seek out. I'm wary of the intangible, could never trust homeopathy. But I appreciate her kindness. And something nags at me: first one eye, now one leg . . .

Shrubs and flowers surround a yellow house with white trim half buried in vegetation: hollyhocks, poppies, clematis, plum and fig trees. There's a fairy-tale quality; we're near a main road, yet the garden is utterly quiet except for the constant singing and rustlings of birds. Enthroned in her wheelchair, wearing a purple shoe today, Phyllis directs me toward the path to the sun-dappled deck. She returns via the house to meet me there. We sit facing each other, and without touching, she hovers her hands above my chest.

Prior to her amputation, Phyllis explains, she and her husband farmed organically. She was a nurse and an artist. One of her clay sculptures, a near life-sized terracotta figure of a young woman, watches us from among some raspberry canes.

I turn as directed while Phyllis passes her hands over every part of me, making small noises of approval or curiosity. Do I feel the energy shift? A kind of warmth? No, but I'm enjoying this all the same. She tells me about her five grandchildren and then, when I ask, the story of how she lost her leg.

It began in a different part of her body: a doctor brushed aside her concerns about a breast lump which ultimately required a total mastectomy, involved a trip to the US, and took three attempts to remove. Years later came a painful swelling in her right thigh. A hiking injury, the doctor thought. She iced, rested; the swelling grew until a Vancouver specialist discovered a hypermalignant growth called pleomorphic liposarcoma and recommended immediate amputation of her entire leg.

"I was lucky. People often resist, but losing my breast made it *way* easier to lose a leg! Even so, it was frightening." On the ferry to Tsawwassen the morning of the surgery, the captain slowed the boat so passengers could watch a pod of orcas. All Phyllis's worries evaporated.

They took the whole leg, right to the hip. Shocking, but better than being dead! After, Phyllis and her husband moved to this house on the edge of town. He tends the garden, feeds the birds. She assists people—women especially—with their health. She uses crutches and a wheelchair. She swims for exercise and reads detective novels to relax.

When Phyllis leans forward, bending double in her chair to rest her hands above my feet, I think I almost feel something, but probably not. She invites me to follow her inside and lie on the sofa, tucks me under a cashmere blanket, orders me to rest, sets a timer for fifteen minutes, and wheels away to another room.

Had I not first met the exquisite cyclops, I might not have accepted Phyllis's offer. I could have missed filtered garden light on a warm afternoon. Missed her kindness and care, missed learning her story. All of which, frankly, feel more sustaining than telehealth.

I hover on the verge of sleep, then close my eyes and walk deep into familiar woods, into the golden light, the air lively with gnats, moths, dragonflies. At the edge of a pool, deep-green and smooth as polished stone, I glimpse my reflection. I, too, have only the one enormous central eye, its iris a blend of blues and greys, of turquoise. A breeze ripples the water, and the eye scatters across the surface, becoming moving patterns of light.

I am in the eye, and I am it. I may have a chance to learn new ways of seeing—of living, even—that I can't yet imagine. I feel a kind of *confidence*. I feel as if I'm on the brink of finding some way to meet the erosion that lies ahead (slow, I hope, but cannot know) of my own physical and mental faculties—

The timer sounds, a faint, tinny tune. It's followed by the soft, sticky squeak of the wheelchair's approach. I open my eyes as Phyllis comes to a halt by the couch.

"Do you feel a bit better?" she asks.

For a long moment, we each study the other. Artfully draped in a cream and lilac dress that complements the purple of her shoe, two-eyed, one-legged, wounded, whole. My new friend, both dreamlike and astonishingly real.

7

~

Neurologists

Their reputations precede them. Brilliant. Arrogant. Kind. Cold. Busy. Too busy. Dedicated. Egomaniac. Forgetful. The possessive *my* is used by those blessed with one who appears to listen and leaves them feeling cared for, even hopeful: "My neurologist is wonderful! Solutions focused. Young, up-to-date, very patient . . . Gay! I was just so lucky to get in when he'd just arrived." Here, a small smile. "I would ask for you, but . . ."

The neurologist may imply a less happy situation, as in "The neurologist gave me a pamphlet and told me there just isn't anything else to try."

Waiting for a referral, and then again for an appointment, I thought again about Anatole Broyard. Suffering from an incurable cancer, he sought to defy its obliterating powers while he still existed by being even more alive than he used to be. He wrote ecstatically, extravagantly, wanted and demanded without limits. His exacting and lengthy list of the qualities he required in a physician began with good taste and style, which would be the last of my concerns. He asserted his need for "a doctor with a sensibility": a physician who appreciated literature, he insisted, giving as suitable examples Anton Chekhov and William Carlos Williams.

"I want him to be my Virgil, leading me through my purgatory or inferno, pointing out the sights as we go," he pronounced, adding, "My ideal doctor would resemble Oliver Sacks."

Who wouldn't want Oliver Sacks, sadly no longer available, a doctor so passionately interested in the qualities of his patients' lives as well as in their fascinating symptoms? The one possible disadvantage of Sacks as doctor applies only to sick writers: if he chose to turn your experience into a brilliant case study, your story would become his and certainly dwarf any of your own attempts.

Broyard also required wit. He insisted he be treated by someone who enjoyed and appreciated him, and he wanted that person to be "not only a talented physician, but a bit of a metaphysician, too." Someone who would "go through my soul." The relationship should be "beautiful in some way." He wants to be seen for the person he is and *transfigured*.

The relationship implied is in no way reciprocal. But I don't feel critical. Broyard was in a hard place. And perhaps some of it was tongue-in-cheek.

As a wealthy American living in New York, Broyard could hire and fire any number of talented specialists, his only limit being the cost and the short time left him. My circumstances are different: a chronic, progressive neurological condition that seems like a much-accelerated aging process with nasty added extras, and a cash-starved not-for-profit public health care system (for which I am grateful). There's little choosing to be done. In any case, my list of requirements has been short from the start: I want my neurologist to be fully informed and competent, and proactive. Or, in the style of Broyard: deeply knowledgeable, experienced, up-to-date, and ready to deploy their skills with every ounce of their ability on my behalf. In such a person I can have confidence and trust they will do the best possible for me. Their manner, within limits, is much less important. It is my experience that expecting one person to satisfy all one's needs rarely works out.

Other items I might hope for? Good communication skills would top the list. I hesitate to insist because they seem rare, as do neurologists. I'm prepared to put effort into compensating for a deficiency. I can interpret and ask for confirmation, politely request further information.

Also on the extras list would be visible compassion, as expressed by a doctor's kindness, ability to listen, and the quality of attention given, qualities Broyard does not specifically mention but could be assuming or considering to be covered by his references to Chekhov and Sacks. Research into the placebo effect shows how powerfully positive expectation can affect the body in real, measurable terms, and a caring manner can significantly affect the amount of positive expectation and trust a patient feels. The same treatment offered with or without attention and compassion will produce different results.

A lack of prejudice, sure! To be seen to some extent for who I am? Wonderful. But while Broyard yearned for perfection, I'll be satisfied with something like Winnicott's good-enough parent. I can turn to other sources for visible caring, connection, and moral support.

But first, an *appointment.*

Broyard would have approved of the physiatrist I was sent to in the middle of my nine-month wait for neurology. Tall and curvaceous, she wore a belted dress in a large, vivid floral print. The fabric looked and sounded like real silk. Her nail polish picked up on its darker pinks and was perfectly applied; I felt sure that beneath the mask her lip colour would likewise coordinate. In the bleak corridors of the Covid-era hospital, these sensuous details stood out. I was at that point so far from dressing with aesthetic considerations in mind that they seemed otherworldly.

She waved me into the room and then to a chair. Made eye contact. What was I here for, she asked, her voice fulsome, almost operatic. But far more valuable than her style was her honesty. "You can rule out MS," she said when the testing was complete. "To me, this seems like Parkinson's, but it's not for me to diagnose. I'm afraid you'll just have to keep waiting for that neurology appointment . . . Are you okay? Can you tell me what I've just said?"

Next, I was offered an appointment with a geriatrician. Desperate, as well as looking at least a decade older than I had the previous year, I had no problem swallowing my pride. He had years of experience with Parkinson's and was prepared to fit me in. His manner was rather subdued, even somewhat withdrawn, but he examined and tested me with great thoroughness, made the diagnosis, and prescribed effective medication.

~

The received wisdom is that neurology attracts the more intellectual, scientific, or philosophically inclined medical students, as well as those who can create good long-term, or longitudinal, relationships with patients who may, because of the nature of their disease, be difficult and headed toward very unpleasant outcomes. It is not a field recommended to the artistically or creatively inclined (no reason given). Yet surely Sacks did more than throw words on a page?

As a realist, I don't think it useful or fair to *expect* perfection. I cannot summon the energy to insist, as some would say I should, on the very best in the land.

Perhaps what enabled Broyard to be so ambitious in his requirements was a generous supply of that vital substance dubbed by Daniel Lieberman the molecule of more. Dopamine.

8

~

Oh, Dopamine!

1

I don't normally do this, but I told two women, innocent strangers I'd only just met, that I have Parkinson's disease. This was on the lookout at the summit of the mountain now known as Mount Maxwell. The far older Hul'q'umi'num' name, *Hwmat'etsum*, means "bent over place"; ironic, given how hard I am trying to avoid that particular Parkinson's posture. The two women wore similar puffy jackets in red and blue and were possibly sisters. How long had it taken me to hike up from the trailhead, the red-jacketed one asked, and both seemed overly impressed with my answer. They, it turned out, had driven almost all the way up. I'm not sure why I felt embarrassed for them, but I did, and so I explained my hike as "doctor's orders." Asked then if I had heart problem, I uttered the terrible word.

"I'm so sorry to hear that," said the older of the two. She treated me to a bright white smile. "But of course, the new medications they have now are just miraculous, aren't they?"

It was a blustery day and more so up there at the top. We were all but shouting at each other. *Yes!* I wished I could wholeheartedly yell. But truth be told, not exactly. Let's say wonderful, then not. Complicated. But as for new—

I was getting cold, and I only had an hour until the next dose, so I loudly agreed and said goodbye.

Carbidopa/levodopa comes in an unassuming small ovoid pill, pale-yellow, tapering in thickness and grooved along the minor axis so you can split it by pressing either side of the groove. I down one and a half of these with 250 millilitres of water four times a day, on a strict schedule which involves not eating for two hours before and one hour after a dose.

The main active ingredient is L-DOPA, from which my brain can make dopamine. L-DOPA has been deployed in treating Parkinson's since the 1960s. So *no*, Mountaintop Woman: this medication is nothing like *new*. And while its benefits may indeed seem miraculous, it has side effects and serious limitations— the biggest being that it does not affect the root cause or halt the disease. Side effects often develop as the disease progresses, which make the drug harder to use. It is still the best or only option for most of us, and PWP live far longer and better than we did before this medication existed. None of the alternatives are cures; all have downsides.

I will likely consume over two thousand of these pills a year, probably more, for the rest of my life. I'm glad that they exist, deeply grateful; yet I will admit to a sliver of resentment at being dependent on an imperfect remedy, and likewise at finding that what's going on in my brain, and how the drug I take works, is difficult to understand.

It melds biochemistry, pharmacology, and neuroscience. I was last involved with chemistry in secondary school. I dropped it as soon as I could, appalled by the requirement to memorize the periodic table. I'm a former novelist prone to invention, daydreaming, dramatization, *and* a person with Parkinson's disease (not known for sharpening one's wits). So I am poorly equipped for the task of explaining it to myself, let alone anyone else. But it seems important to try.

Dopamine, named from the description of its molecular structure—3,4-dihydroxyphenethylamine— is now understood to be vital to life as we know it. It is manufactured by a small number of specialized neurons huddled in that ancient part of the midbrain that seems to be the source of all our problems, the substantia nigra. It's a two-step process. First, an amino acid, tyrosine (known as one of the "building blocks of life"), is converted into L-DOPA. From that, with the assistance of a particular enzyme (these are proteins that help speed up chemical reactions in our bodies), dopamine is made and latches onto the cells that need it.

It took much of the last century to establish that the brains of people with Parkinson's no longer make the amount of dopamine needed to enable both voluntary and involuntary movements and that this is the cause of tremors, weakness, shuffling gait, and so on. Early-twentieth-century pharmacologists, however, were not interested in dopamine, seeing it as a mere stage on the way to the manufacture of adrenalin, also known as epinephrine, which they were very keen to investigate.

Progress was therefore slow: levodopa had been isolated from fava bean plants in 1913, but the enzyme needed to make it into dopamine was not stumbled upon until 1938; understanding what it was, where it was, and what it did took yet further decades.

Arvid Carlsson first published on the topic in November 1957; by that time others were interested too. Katharine Montagu had published on the same topic in August 1957. Carlsson, who would be the recipient of the 2000 Nobel Prize in Physiology or Medicine, is credited with discovering dopamine in the human brain and kickstarting the subsequent rush of understanding as to its role in enabling effective movement. Confirmation that dopamine deficiency was indeed the cause of Parkinson's motor symptoms led to the use of levodopa (L-DOPA) as a dopamine replacement during the late 1960s. L-DOPA was licensed in the US in 1970 and since then has remained the main treatment for Parkinson's. During the past five decades, it has become clear that many non-motor Parkinson's symptoms are also affected by Lieberman's "molecule of more."

"That no better drug for Parkinson's disease has been found than the first one discovered 40 years ago is a vanishingly rare pharmacological phenomenon," Alison Abbott wrote in *Nature* magazine in 2010—already fifteen years ago. So, Dear Woman on the Mountaintop, please note that even scientists acknowledge that better treatment for Parkinson's disease is slow to emerge and *not one bit new*, despite the huge amount of research that continues to investigate possible causes of the disease and its mechanisms in the hope of finding new ways to alleviate, prevent, or cure it.

What seems to be emerging is a picture of an extraordinarily complicated disease with an ever-growing list of symptoms. It affects many more areas of the brain than initially thought. The sheer variety of ways in which it presents and in which symptoms cluster leads some neurologists to think that what we now call Parkinson's is several, or many, related diseases. It seems unlikely that researchers will find a single cause; those offered so far include heredity, exposure to chemical pollutants, and bacterial infection in the gut. Hypotheses as to helpful new treatments, when tested, raise yet further questions to be investigated. Because the disease is so multifaceted and complicated, our new knowledge seems to spread laterally rather than focus and lead to an answer (or answers). There has been more progress in terms of early detection than in treatment or cure.

Clearly, though, what is taking place in Parkinson's-afflicted brains like mine is unpleasant, to consider as well as to experience. Vital parts are dying because of a "misfolded" protein called alpha-synuclein. It accumulates, gathers into clumps, and kills off the relatively tiny but hugely important cluster of dopamine-producing neurons in the substantia nigra. There are ten different subtypes of cells within the substantia nigra, and only very recently have scientists identified the relatively rare one responsible for dopamine production.

Misfolded? How? By whom? Images of crumpled laundry and veiled robot-nuns come to mind, but all I really need to know is that some kind of error in the chemical manufacture of these proteins has lethal consequences.

Why does the protein start misfolding? This is not yet clear, but at the time of writing, some scientists suspect a particular kind of gut bacteria is responsible for making that happen, while others suspect the vagus ("wandering, meandering") nerve might provide a route for the misfolds to travel to the brain. So, a PWP is bound to ask, Could a simple targeted antibiotic blitz, followed by colonic irrigation and an easy-peasy fecal transplant of benevolent gut bacteria resolve this whole sad mess?

Just imagine the parties! But no, we're not there yet. Studies continue.

How do the misfolded, clumping proteins do the killing? Starvation, suffocation? Clumping sounds both fluffy and sticky, like dumplings. If anyone does know, they are not making it clear. In any case, this neuron-killing process, parthanatos, named after Thanatos, the Greek god of death, sets off an inflammatory response that causes further mayhem and yet more brain-cell death.

Dopamine-producing neurons in our brains don't heal or replace themselves. The result of the slaughter is a chronic and increasingly devastating shortage of brain dopamine. By the time symptoms become obvious and someone can no longer sign their name and is shuffling and shaking their way to diagnosis, as much as 80 percent of their dopamine-producing neurons have died.

What happens to the dead neurons? Do they fester in place, causing more problems? Are they somehow reabsorbed? Ugh. I really don't need to know.

2

It may have been described by Oliver Sacks and others as seemingly miraculous, but L-DOPA also has a reputation as a "pharmacologist's nightmare." Alison Abbott calls it "a most difficult molecule to control therapeutically, thanks to its inconveniently short biological half-life, physicochemical cussedness and poorly understood pharmacodynamic interaction with disease progression. . . . It looks small and innocent, but has an incompliant chemistry and unhelpful metabolism."

Moving the rather helpful but inconvenient and *physicochemically cussed* levodopa from the digestive system into the blood and from there into the brain is not a simple process. In keeping with its awkward nature, it is only absorbed in a small area of the intestine just below the stomach. This is why we are advised not to eat close to a dose. And L-DOPA is not an independent traveller. Once it has reached the absorption zone, special transporter proteins are required to carry it through the wall of the small intestine into the bloodstream. I'm imagining these transporters as sherpas, wiry and fit; the cumbersome, overdressed traveller levodopa roped to them as they make their way up scree-strewn slopes to some kind of narrow tunnel from the far end of which they will launch themselves into the red torrent.

Once in the bloodstream, levodopa begins to degrade, quickly becoming unusable. At the blood-brain barrier, the levodopa is again assisted (this time perhaps by calm but steely-eyed, stylishly dressed officials?) across the border (here I envisage a narrow, high-tech checkpoint manned by soldiers and sniffer dogs) and then on in a self-driving vehicle at alarming speed through complicated pinky-grey tunnels, across multiple branching intersections, in and down to a sudden halt for an automated ID check at the dark portal to the even darker substantia nigra where, exhausted and quite possibly terrified, levodopas must find the highly specialized striatal dopaminergic nerve terminals, with which they must in some chemical fashion "bond."

It's not clear to me (nor so far as I can see to anyone else) exactly how, given the bad conditions in the substantia nigra, the much-travelled and perhaps exhausted L-DOPA manages to find the relevant enzyme and connect to the correct receptors in the striatal dopaminergic nerve terminals. My diminished imagination fails me, but perhaps envisage these terminals as something like an EV charger?

Somehow, at last, the substance we all want, usable dopamine, becomes available. Orders once again travel swiftly and efficiently along the nerves, perhaps rather like little LED lights chasing each other along a transparent tube, and lo and behold! Rigid musculature relaxes, tremors calm, and with our faces mobile and expressive once more, we stride out into the world, loosely swinging our arms and feeling relatively capable, indeed, almost normal. Blow trumpets! Sing "Hallelujah"!

Under good conditions, all this transportation and conversion takes between twenty and sixty minutes, and then you have a period of relief. Mine currently lasts four hours, though it began nearer six. A dose tends to peak and then diminish.

I need these small, gritty, yellow pills to live what is called well: pretty much normally at least some of the time. Even so, misfolded proteins continue to gather and clump in my brain; dopamine-producing neurons in my brain's black stuff continue to keel over and die. As the disease progresses (worsens), the effects of L-DOPA become noticeably less consistent and more likely to include unwanted extras, the best known of these being medication-induced dyskinesia (involuntary writhing movements).

Most PWP end up increasing their consumption of L-DOPA to obtain something increasingly inferior to the initial response.

This may sound familiar, but what would happen to me if I stopped taking my medication is not the same as an addict's withdrawal, during which, ideally, the swings between drug-exaggerated high and consequent exaggerated low gradually return to a pre-addiction condition of balance (homeostasis) and lesser range. Rather it would be a confrontation with a new reality, with what I have unknowingly become due to disease progression. To avoid this occurring, I carry several days' supply with me at all times.

Medication is a treasured relief, but also, now, an unwelcome reminder that I'm running out of juice. Of time. As the neurologist said, "It works until it doesn't."

End of story? Swallow them down, and go gathering rosebuds while ye may? Not quite yet. In keeping with L-DOPA's cussed chemistry, there are a few more complications. That dopamine is vital to the regulation of movement—not just the more obvious walking, running, swimming, and so on but also speech, sewing, beating eggs, typing, writing, and even the vital involuntary movements that occur beyond our awareness, like gut motility—is increasingly well-known.

Less familiar is the understanding that a lack of dopamine (and of other "feel-good" hormones and neurotransmitters) affects not just the physical, muscular part of carrying out an action, but the motivation that makes it possible for it to occur in the first place.

3

Most of the dopamine-deprived succumb to some extent to what my friend and fellow PWP Linda calls the "Parkinson's triumvirate": lethargy, apathy, depression. The way Linda puts it is that 1) you feel too tired and can't be bothered to start a project, 2) you don't much care that you're too tired to get anything done, and then 3) you feel down because you don't care and are getting nothing done. And of course, you can't be bothered to do anything about that either. Not that this is her problem, Linda hastens to add, slyly. No. She's just enjoying the irony.

Months later, telling me about her visit to a counsellor, she makes it clear that she is not depressed, not at all. She wanted to set something up for the future, just in case.

A former freelance editor and writer who used to travel the world in the course of her work for international commissions and environmental organizations, Linda once researched and wrote a book in twelve weeks. The volume and complexity of the frequently intricate and collaborative work she accomplished now seem extraordinary to her. Five years into Parkinson's, running the support group and writing summaries of its monthly meetings have to satisfy the powerful desire she has always had to serve by doing work that improves, rather than harms, the way we live and how we relate to the more-than-human world we inhabit.

She can't imagine how she did what she used to do. Worse than that, given government inaction in response to the climate emergency and rampant inequity, it can seem as if all that passionate conviction and all that work—those meetings, those deadlines met, those chapters and reports written or edited—were an utter waste of time. Added to that, as she sees the worsening situation of others in the support group, it's impossible not to be acutely aware of what lies ahead for her on the medical front. Even now, she seems to be lurching from one fall or health crisis to the next and has had to give up driving. Following one meeting, during a long attempt to buckle her seat belt in my car, Linda confided that she could see a point when her life might be too horrible to endure and admitted to both herself and me that yes, she was depressed, right now. She decided to try the antidepressant her doctor had offered. To her surprise, and heaven knows exactly how, it works.

So-called mood changes affect most PWP to some degree and go beyond routine depression. In addition to Linda's lethargy, apathy, and depression triumvirate, there is something called the Parkinson's personality which includes obsessiveness, inflexibility, anxiety, pessimism, shyness, even a "persistent sense of dread and foreboding." None of these are attractive traits, and for some, they begin years before diagnosis. Inflexibility? No. But I can attest to increasing anxiety and pessimism over the past decade. Given the state of our planet and ourselves, it seems a reasonable response—but not so much when it also shows up, as I must admit it did prior to the antidepressants, in the obsessive checking of travel and other plans.

In the later stages of the disease, personality changes may be so severe as to make the sufferer seem to their family and intimate associates "like another person": not only depressed but intermittently aggressive, withdrawn, self-focused, or unreasonably demanding. "Belligerent and insensitive" was how one now-widowed carer described to me her husband's increasingly frequent "odd spells" during the final months of his life. She had been drawn to him at least in part because of his lively mind and sweet disposition, which made this change seem particularly cruel.

By now, it is perhaps no surprise to learn that the lethargy, apathy, and depression Linda speaks of are thought to result, just like movement symptoms, from dopamine deficiency.

According to Lieberman and Long in *The Molecule of More*, it's now understood that dopamine is released when we encounter things that are notable or, as neurologists express it, salient to us, especially if what we encounter is in some way new or unexpected. When we encounter potential life sustainers or enhancers, particularly those that are new to us, dopamine floods us with a potent blend of curiosity, desire, excitement, anticipation: in a word, arousal, which pushes us to pursue and act in order to obtain what we desire.

Both motive and muscle are needed to get anything done, and dopamine, it seems, fuels them both, if we have enough of it. We who are deficient tend to be less engaged and less motivated. We do less, connect less with others, and feel increasingly depressed.

It's the same for other animals: according to one study, starved rats deprived of brain dopamine will not retrieve food placed even a few inches away from where they sit.

Of course, many human desires cannot be easily attained and are not a matter of simply reaching out a hand to pluck fruit from the tree. Satisfying some of our needs and wants requires mental as well as physical effort: visualization, planning, strategy, and co-operation with others may be required.

In this, too, dopamine is involved. In a part of the brain called the prefrontal cortex (the outer layer of the bit before the front), it plays a vital role in terms of enabling the high-level set of skills collectively known as executive function. Executive function is what enables us to generate ideas, organize thoughts; to work alone or with others for days, months, or years to change or create something. Self-control, imagination, reflection, prediction, strategizing, goal-setting, organization, problem-solving: dopamine has fingers in all those pies.

Recent research confirms that dopamine-producing neurons in the ventral tegmental area (underside covering), or VTA, located in another part of the midbrain and responsible for these much-prized prefrontal executive functions, degenerate and die at a much higher rate in PWP than is normal for the general population. A scrap of comfort can perhaps be found in the detail that they die somewhat more slowly than those in the substantia nigra.

Dopamine, as well as allowing us to feel desire and take physical action to satisfy it, enables us to use our brains to plan and our hands and tools to create new realities. New is important. Researchers have demonstrated that when we are faced with something of value but routinely available, we and other animals may still engage with or consume it if it is around, but there will be no dopamine release. Items that provoke dopamine release tend to be new or newly relevant, especially attractive or challenging, rather than familiar good things.

For some PWP, the distressing symptom cluster related to loss of executive function, tactfully described in waiting room leaflets as "cognitive changes," are the disease's crowning humiliation. These include drastically reduced productivity and a decreased ability to organize, solve complex problems, and/or multi-task. Those, like my friend Stan, who have used these skills in work they were passionately committed to, find this loss to be at the heart of the sense of diminishment they and many PWP feel.

More than a decade into the disease, Stan suffers from many alarming and disabling movement-related symptoms, including periods of festination when he has to run rather than walk and can only stop himself by running into something, such as a wall or kitchen counter. He falls often and frequently in dangerous environments. Despite this, he feels that neurologists and researchers focus too narrowly on physical symptoms while neglecting the mental and psychological aspects of the disease such as decline in executive powers and depression. He battles both.

As a lawyer who worked over many decades in criminal, aboriginal, and other forms of law, Stan was used to a very high level of function and was passionately motivated in his work. At one time he represented Ann Hansen, one of the "Squamish Five," who was prosecuted in the early 1980s for a variety of charges related to direct action taken against, among others, a BC Hydro substation, a chain of pornography stores, and Litton Industries in Toronto. (Litton was intending to supply parts for American-made cruise missiles.) Later, he represented the families of mistreated prisoners.

There was in his work a focus on the underdog and on political challenges to the status quo. It was an absorbing, successful career and gave him great satisfaction and sense of purpose. He was used to being confident, articulate, effective, and purposeful both on his own account and as part of a team—and used to feeling he was making a significant and meaningful contribution.

About ten years ago, at a time when Stan was working on workers' compensation claims, peculiar symptoms began to intrude: an involuntary side-to-side movement of his head, for example. "My colleagues assumed I was disagreeing with everything they said! They'd comment; I had to explain. Then I started to fall asleep, even in the middle of a sentence, talking with a client." His memory grew unreliable. His speech slurred. And he noticed a reduced ability to organize, whether it was the flow of work or ideas. This improved once he got treatment, but only temporarily.

"There was the levodopa honeymoon, perhaps four or five years, but it's a distant memory now . . . I knew," he continues, and his soft voice and even tone, so very much at odds with what he is saying, accrues a kind of negative expressiveness of its own, "I knew that I couldn't offer the same level of service. It wasn't right to continue." At sixty-four, he resigned as partner from the practice he had joined at the age of twenty-six.

"That was maybe . . . five or six years ago. A big loss. I'd certainly have continued otherwise . . . I still miss it. It's one of the things I miss most. Being in charge of things. Organizing. It's gone. And I miss my voice . . ." Of course. A lawyer's voice is a vital tool, an instrument used in court to elicit trust and influence others' thoughts and emotions. Now we can barely make out what he's saying. That Stan is depressed is scarcely a surprise.

Like Linda, I take an antidepressant and I have done so since all this began. I am certainly aware of my own cognitive changes, though it seems that few others notice them. Even when medication returned some of the physical ability to write and type, I did not think in the same way.

I abandoned my half-written novel, having neither the stamina nor the motivation needed to complete such a complicated large-scale project, and little interest in a topic that had fascinated me before. There was a strange hush where all that passion, drive, and absorbed activity used to be, as if the bees had left the hive.

As I and countless other creative writing instructors tell our creative writing students, desire drives the story. *Until that changes,* an inner voice now adds. You can bring only essentials to this other country, the kingdom of the sick.

Does dopamine or our lack of it make us who we are? It certainly affects many aspects of our behaviour and capabilities. How you see this depends on how rigidly you define or characterize yourself. For sure, I'm reluctant to accept that the way I think, feel, and behave is the result of an imbalance in biochemistry, and not in some way "me." It seems reductive. I'd like at least to cling to the notion that in some way my history of interactions and experiences might affect how the chemistry expresses itself, even when it is pathological, and likewise regarding how I cope with what it delivers.

I remember hiking furiously up my favourite mountain, failing to push past tears. I stopped to sit on a rock, gave in. I reminded myself that it's not just me: age or injury forces most people to confront the question as to what to do or be *instead*. Losing a vocation or profession is terrible, but far from the most frightening thing a person faces. I reminded myself of other people, relationships, causes, and activities that I care about, but my heart still ached.

At the broad, steep slope below the summit, where the giant Douglas firs soar, there, in sudden coolness, in the alert silence between the big trees, it came to me, softly as a breeze-blown cobweb, that I was making an all-or-nothing assumption. That yes, I continue to be exiled from the imaginary realm. My brain and body are changing. What I can or want to do, with words in particular, is bound to be different to what I did before. There is no point in striving for the previous now-impossible thing. Do what's possible.

Let's say that for a while at least there may be something new. Observe what is in front of me, this new reality unfolding, open a window so others can see themselves or come to understand how it is to go through these changes. I can make a sentence work. So: write one, then another. If I use the abilities I still possess and work patiently with the material and my changed brain, I may succeed in making something meaningful in response to my losses and create, despite the obstacles, something of value that connects with others.

I thanked the trees and took the next trail down.

~

Since learning a little about how vital dopamine is to human and animal life, I've become acutely sensitive to other people's dopamine levels. I may be fooling myself, but they seem easy to detect. At the one end of the spectrum is the subdued, low-energy mode of most in the PWP support group. At the other is the dopaminergic personality. These creative, curious, exploratory people have plenty (but not a dangerous excess) of the substance we PWP lack. Busy with ideas, relationships, and projects, they fizz with energy, don't want to stop until the job is done, and when it is, they are thinking already of how to start something new or better. Some are extroverts with loud voices and big gestures; others are more introverted and intense. The common ground is a gravitation toward the new, a need to change—improve, they feel—how things are. Paint the house, campaign, write, rewrite, build, produce.

Encountering highly dopaminergic types, particularly in a group, I feel overwhelmed by the intoxicating rush of desire and creative energy flowing through them, and I remember—sadly, and jealously—how I used to be one too.

Some PWP still do achieve a huge amount, but comparisons with others, like comparisons with our own previous capacities, are not helpful. Afflicted celebrities like Michael J. Fox deserve admiration and gratitude but do of course have the advantage of considerable resources and massive support systems, as well as top-notch care.

This disease, a black hole, absorbs energy and capacity. Under its influence, we lose our voices, become demotivated stick-at-homes who observe and note rather than imagine, persist rather than live, coordinate and organize only on a very small scale. Ironically, this comes at a time when much of what we are advised to do for ourselves to slow down disease progression requires huge amounts of motivation.

While the yellow pills work, it is possible to feel like a decent facsimile of our former selves. But there's no better solution to reduced capacity or complete lack of stamina—that sudden feeling of utter depletion—than to accept it and find workarounds. Squeeze out a few miserly drops of willpower, ask others to push and encourage us, trick or argue ourselves into getting started, and endlessly forgive ourselves for being what we are becoming. Break activities into stages, return time and time again to a task previously completed in an hour or so. It's very slow and we will achieve differently and almost certainly less than before, but it's not nothing . . .

That comes later.

Can I make a virtue of this necessity?

Is there a way to reframe dopamine deprivation as an interesting challenge? Could it be that this experience offers—or forces upon me—a new perspective, one from which I'll be able to appreciate the benefits of doing less, or even nothing at all? That I will finally learn to enjoy or at least fully accept things as they are, rather than what I'm in the process of making out of them?

9

~

My Neurologist

I'd almost come to accept my medicated limbo as a permanent state when the call came: a virtual appointment with a neurologist the following week. Now here he was on my screen: a confident man at the young end of middle age, short-haired, bespectacled, alert, healthy-looking.

I apologized for the lack of visible symptoms: a joke of sorts, admittedly lame. He smiled briefly, then leaned back a little in his ultra-high-end ergonomic chair, hands palms down on the tidy desk spread out in front of him.

"We have lots of good information in the file," he said, "but take me through it in your own words."

I kept it brief but dense, leaning heavily on physical facts and memorized dates. I'd had practice by then.

"Yes," he said at the end, with a firmness that I guessed might be his particular way of communicating with sick and possibly impaired patients. And if so, I wouldn't let it bother me—after months of prevarication from many other professionals, clarity was a gift. "Yes. I can confirm that you have Parkinson's disease. You must have been developing this well before you noticed the anosmia—perhaps for a decade or even two—but you were fit and healthy and your brain and body found workarounds. We call that early period the *prodrome*." An appropriately ominous word. Did I have questions?

"People kept telling me Parkinson's doesn't happen *fast*, but it did. It has happened very fast," I told him. "One symptom piled onto the next over a few months. So could that viral heart infection I had just before—"

"Yes," he said, again emphatically. "Another illness can exacerbate progression. Because you are weakened, a thing you have coped with suddenly becomes difficult to correct or ignore."

"It was terrifying," I told him, to which he didn't immediately say *yes*. The pause may or may not have been some kind of acknowledgment on his part. I willed my eyes to stop watering. This was relief, not self-pity. It seemed very important to have my painfully and painstakingly acquired sense of the story of this thing confirmed by a professional. This confirmation was all at once a good thing, a terrible thing, and a mere bureaucratic necessity. Now that I had it, I realized, staring at the image of "my" neurologist on my screen, its importance would quite rapidly diminish.

"Yes. But now," he waved aside my past terrors, "you are responding to treatment and doing well. Are there other questions?"

Medication. I've read about other drugs being used but met only one person doing so. Why a carbidopa/levodopa combination (a decarboxylase inhibitor and a central nervous system agent respectively) as opposed to, say, a monoamine oxidase type B inhibitor or a dopamine receptor agonist like pramipexole? They are all different ways of achieving the same result—that is, making more dopamine available. Some of the others slow the breakdown or the reabsorption of dopamine and can be used alongside carbidopa/levodopa. Some are not yet authorized here or are not covered by pharmacare. He shrugs, adds, "In my opinion, you're highly unlikely to get a better outcome than you have. But we can look into alternatives if you want to experiment."

Clear. Fairly patient, though I sense he would not react well to anything he considered to be foolish, or to outright dissent.

"Roughly how long will this treatment work for me?"

"Five good years is typical, though it can be considerably more, or less. Unfortunately, it becomes a matter of increased dosing and diminishing returns. You are losing vital neurons, and it doesn't stop that happening. Nor do the alternatives."

"So should I begin with the absolute minimum? Will that postpone side effects and make some kind of good effect last longer?"

"I wouldn't say that. The way we put it now is that some of the more serious issues that have been associated with long-term use are actually due to the progress of the disease. People taking this medication are living longer and more normal lives. Nothing is gained by taking less than you need to feel as functional as possible."

"I wouldn't say that" and "The way we put it now" seem less categorical than his previous simple affirmatives, but I let it pass. Best not to seem difficult. Instead, another lame joke and another quick flicker of a smile:

"So, should I take a bit more and feel even better?"

"You seem pretty well! Maintain the current dose. And keep up the exercise . . ."

Not a hint of transfiguration. No evidence of poetry-reading. Effective fact delivery, albeit with few visible signs of empathy. But perhaps he's found that calmly sticking to the facts works best. He must see an awful lot of us, all headed to hell in a handbasket. It went well, I tell those who enquire.

10

~

Be Here Now

Parkinson's and other neurodegenerative diseases render us more susceptible to stress, explains Magali, the younger of the two presenters of "Non-motor Symptoms: Stress Management for Parkinson's," which is the subject of her current research. The "stress hormone" cortisol makes our symptoms worse. Things you didn't use to think of as stressful become so—talking in a small group of friends or one-on-one with a new person, for example. Even just explaining something to the teller at the bank. Leaving the house. Unfamiliar journeys, however short. Driving. You might find your tremor returns, your voice vanishes, or you start dystonic writhing on the spot. Some may experience more freezing in place, a worsening of balance. Feelings of panic. Does this feel familiar? Magali suggests a show of hands: unanimous.

She passes the presentation over to the therapist, Julia, a jolly, rosy-cheeked woman of middle age. What then to do? Some stress is an inevitable and necessary part of life, but frequent or constant stress is undesirable. We do what we can to avoid it, for example, by letting our friends know in advance how we may be feeling, rather than compounding stress by trying to conceal the situation, though that's not always possible.

For PWP, avoiding social or travel stresses by staying in and talking to no one is a clearly bad idea, likely to result in isolation and depression. Julia has two main recommendations: learning simple on-the-spot mindfulness techniques to reduce stress that is already occurring or about to, along with—I knew it was coming—a regular meditation practice.

~

I borrowed several library books for my first, teen-aged attempt at meditation, back in the 1970s. I'd heard meditation could make dramatic changes to a person's consciousness without being dangerous, and was keen to explore it. I remember one of the books as *Be Here Now*, and how I liked the three-syllable title; years later, prompted by listening to some old taped letters of mine from this time prior to archiving them, I could not find the meditation guide I thought was in that particular book. But here is what I recall:

You sat with your legs folded in a lotus position, your hands upward on your knees, your back straight, your chin tucked, and the crown of your head skyward, *see diagram*. You were supposed to close your eyes, but given the need to read the rest of the instructions, I had to keep opening and closing with almost stroboscopic effect. Learning a complicated meditation method from a book is not ideal, but our library's selection of cassette tapes was meagre.

You had to imagine a "being of pure light and love" sitting in a lotus flower on a lake. I enjoyed this, but then you were supposed to picture him—*him?* After the interesting open-endedness of *being*, the specificity was a jolt; I had to reimagine. The next step was to have the image floating just slightly above your eye level—but your eyes were closed, so how did that happen? You were to look up at an angle of thirty degrees, *see diagram*. Should I use a protractor? If so, I'd have to keep my eyes open, find it in my school bag, start over. I decided against this.

Having set up the mental imagery, the next step was to close my left nostril by pressing with my right forefinger and breathe out through my right nostril, visualizing the air expelled as a *dark-red cloud consisting of all bodily attachments and diseases.* (*If only!* I think now.) Back then, I had no diseases and no idea what the author meant by bodily attachments, but it didn't sound good and the idea of that dark-red cloud full of nasty bodily stuff was simultaneously disgusting and hilarious. Unable to laugh and throw up at the same time, I gave up.

For the next attempt, I checked out a book that specified only a warm room and comfortable position, along with closed eyes, steady breath (no nostril closing), and calmly labelling thoughts in order to disconnect from them.

Since our house was always cold, I ran a bath, added Badedas, eased in, stretched out, and relaxed into the warmth. Eyes closed, I made sure to breathe deeply. For several minutes, familiar fractal-like geometric patterns danced behind my eyelids, one morphing hypnotically into the next—something that now and then happened when I was very tired and closed my eyes. Calmly, I labelled my curious thoughts as to what caused these patterns, and soon the patterns, though *not* the thoughts, diminished and faded leaving me with a dark background of soft, slowly but constantly shifting cloud-like shapes. A shifting nothingness.

After a while, I began to detect in this nothingness a reddish tinge that reminded me of the cloud of attachments and diseases. My eyes sprang open.

It struck me how very much I liked to see things, more than that, to really *look at them*. To look and look and look. At steam thickening the air. At how the window and the mirrors cloud over, then weep; at my own breasts and nipples, poking through the thin coating of Badedas bubbles on top of the water, a kind of foam blanket that was pulled right up to my neck. I even liked to look at the bathroom itself, achingly familiar as it was, at the watery-blue tiles to my right, a school of hand-painted fish—herring, probably—swimming through elegantly grouped clusters of seaweed, caught in a perpetual collision course with a school of plump-looking angelfish travelling left to right behind the taps. Between these tiles and the sloping, attic-y ceiling stretched an expanse of wallpaper put up by my father not very long ago, blue and white mixed together like a summer sky—

I knew I should not be looking at it but continued to do so.

Why the insistence on closed eyes for meditation? Did seeing make you think? Or was the liking of it the problem, an attachment? There must be a reason, but so far the book had not revealed it. Inhale slowly, hold, and exhale even more slowly, it had said. Try to be *aware, in your body, in the moment.* (This was interesting and seemed quite a turnaround from the previous method.) I understood a moment was a very tiny bit of time so it should have been doable. But then I coughed and both bathwater and bubble-scum picked up the movement, quivered into ripples that reflected, between the mounds of bubbles, broken pieces of the white globe of the ceiling lamp. Soon it all subsided, flattened, was gone: an ordinary thing, but amazing, too—I was glad not to have missed it and felt vindicated for slackening off on the closed eyes and calm labelling of thoughts.

I then began thinking of more *obviously* extraordinary visual things—of Salvador Dalí's melting clocks and distorted flesh, his surfaces crawling with ants and flies, elephants on stilts—wondering did he see those strange forms, hallucinate them even, *before* he painted them, or were they invented in *the now*, on the canvas, in some kind of collaboration between it, him, and the sable or bristle tip, Salvador perhaps twirling his moustache as he pushed the paint around, creating something doodle-like and yet real-seeming in the extreme? According to my art teacher, white-haired, brightly smocked Fiona Montrose, art was all about *looking* and then *rendering the world* and the *way the light falls.* I knew rendering was *not* rending, but still, it was an unattractive word that can also be used about boiling bones to make glue. Miss Montrose had taken our class to the Tate but would not share her own opinion of Dalí because she wanted us to think for ourselves and complete the worksheet.

I wrote that I did not positively like the paintings, but they were hard to forget.

What, then, to make of Uri Geller's bent spoons? Dalí made real in at least three dimensions! My physics teacher said psychokinesis was a ludicrous fiction, merely a spectacle for TV. If this spoon-bender was genuine, he'd let scientists wire him up and study him. My mother wondered why he didn't use his mind power to do something useful. I wondered if there could be forces as yet unknown that simply couldn't be measured with existing instruments. Wasn't it possible that physics might need to adjust its laws to account for an extraordinary phenomenon?

Thoughts . . .

I rose shivering from the tub, tugged the giant towel, pale-blue background with swans in white, from the heated chrome-pipe towel rail that Dad had recently installed. Wrapped in swans, I settled on the mat with my back against the side of the bath, stared at the three gleaming chrome rails on the wall a few feet away and thought how amazing it would be to bend them.

The idea was irresistible. I tucked my then highly bendable legs into the half-lotus position, rearranged the towel-cape, stared at the gleaming metal: a blend of silver and white and black that included my own reflection stretched and distorted like one of Dalí's melted clocks. *Bend*, I mentally instructed the middle of the three rails. (It was at eye level, so no degrees of elevation were involved.) My jaw loosened. *Bend*, I told the rail again. I managed to merely note and then relax the smile that yearned to form. *Bend . . . breathe . . . bend, breathe, bend . . .* Going right off script, feeling my way by instinct, I pictured a cloud of minute pearly particles pulsing around my body and then gathering where, according to *Be Here Now*, my third eye resided. I visualized the pulsing particles beaming out from the front of my brain toward the chrome rail, which was a far more substantial thing than a cheap spoon and might not have been the best choice for a total beginner. I knew I mustn't think—which funnily enough was easier now that I had a task to achieve. Or was visualizing thinking too? In any case,

I pictured the subatomic particles, a sort of cosmic dust vibrating in harmony, a wave of them pouring out through my chest and the pupil of my imagined third eye and wrapping itself around the rail. I imagined a deep humming, then heard myself making the same sound as I exhaled. I pulled the air in, out, in, out, willed the pipe to *bend, bend, bend* . . . What madness! But I felt strangely calm, sure that I was right on the verge of being in control of both towel rail and self.

Breathe, bend, bend, bend. Breathe, bend, bend, bend . . . And then— Was it curving downward—as if a section of it were softening, stretching? It *was*! Yet when I reached out to touch, the rail remained straight and rigid, as well as scalding hot—and I, light-headed, chilly, with pins and needles in both feet, was right back *here, now*, in the ordinary bathroom, the mirrors and windows streaming with condensation.

~

During the five decades since these early experiments, there have been many other abandoned meditation attempts, including one in my mid-twenties that lasted for several weeks.

It's startling to realize that at least half of our friends are meditators of one kind or another. One is a Zen master. At a potluck early in the year, Richard and I were the only two there not practising. When conversation gravitated to the topic, we sat in our chairs, silent, smiles affixed, while others enthusiastically shared snippets of wisdom, talked about a retreat some planned to attend, spoke rhapsodically about zazen, sitting meditation, and how many hours of it the retreat provided.

We all laughed when I took advantage of a moment of silence to confess to a detestation of sitting straight-backed and motionless on the floor, alone or in a group and with or without a folded blanket under my boney buttocks. This prompted the Zen master to confess in turn that long ago, as a novice, he had found ways to mitigate discomfort when sitting for long periods by making tiny, surreptitious shifts and stretches under cover of his voluminous black robe, despite having been given the traditional instruction to accept or disconnect from the discomfort rather than adjust to relieve it. Everyone enjoyed this admission too.

I can see that acceptance and disconnection learned by sitting on a hard floor would be good training for enduring far worse things. I can at least imagine the benefits of suspending the torrent of mental activity some call "monkey mind," of having a break, a deep rest—or even making a first step on the way to an utterly different state of being, the very thing that first drew the teenaged me to select *Be Here Now* from the library shelves. I would be delighted to experience a sense of merging with the universe, but fully understand that that is the outcome of years of practice and not for the casual taking of lazy non-starters like me. And of course, since diagnosis, the value of living in what is known as *the now* is very clear to me, since, as Emily Dickinson put it in poem 1741, "That it will never come again / Is what makes life so sweet."

Even so, I confess that despite scientific evidence that particular brain activity patterns are connected to the feeling of deep, profoundly restorative relaxation experienced by dedicated practitioners, I have so far been incapable of devoting regular time to overcome my discomfort and quibbles in the cause of developing and benefitting from regular meditation practice. Richard has not even felt the need to try.

It may be that the ability to experience *the now*, the ongoing present via the calm, aware, connective state that meditators describe, will become more accessible to me if I can find less formal routes to it. For example, resting on the hot rock of our favourite beach after a swim, hearing the slip and slap of waves on the shore. Or walking, especially in the woods. Listening to birds, the wind in the trees. Eating. Performing a monotonous outdoor task, such as cleaning garlic or stacking firewood. I know, I know—these examples are situation dependent, whereas a lifelong meditator can sit down anywhere, breathe, detach from irritating bodily sensations and monkey mind, and shift gear into alert nowness within a few breaths. Those who have practised enough may not even have to sit.

So yes, when Julia's presentation ends, I will sign up in the hope of being able to learn a twenty-minute meditation technique. I will try again, and likely fail again. And meanwhile I remind myself that there is no need for musical accompaniment, podcast, or audiobook when I weed the garden. That it is enough—more—to just be where I am: squatting in the dirt, pulling weeds, and calmly noting the wind in the trees. The busyness of worms and larvae in the soil. The sun's warmth on my neck. The gurgling of my guts.

11

~

Chronic

We are, for good evolutionary reasons, disgusted by substances that could make us sick—including, of course, our own bodily wastes and particularly what was known in my distant UK childhood as "number two." All the senses, but especially that of smell, are involved in this experience of revulsion.

Dealing with our own excreta is normally a private affair. We fear exposure, other people's repulsion, and we rarely want to communicate about this part of our lives. When we need to, it's difficult. How to find middle ground between baby talk, medicalization, and curse word? Doo-doo, shite, crap, feces, turd . . . *Poop* is the cheery North American term. So how to fully convey, without repelling the reader and provoking cries of "Too much information," the banal reality that's become a source of mental as well as physical suffering for so many struggling with Parkinson's and other conditions, too: the deeply humiliating and ongoing struggle we engage in to rid ourselves of our own shit?

James Joyce, coprophiliac and far from squeamish in his private life, included an outhouse scene in *Ulysses*. In it, Leopold Bloom defecates at leisure while reading a magazine, relishing the control he has over the act, brought about by a dose of cascara he took the day before to overcome a "mild case" of constipation. He notes his own "rising smell" without judgment and, given the nature of the man, could well be enjoying it.

Joyce used to be pretty much the only example. Now, depictions of defecation and even constipation are quite common. They even may be very detailed and lengthy, to the point that Norwegian writer Karl Ove Knausgård has been accused of "gratuitous attention to detail" in this respect, his defence as quoted by Ian MacDougall in a *Paris Review* article being that in such scenes he is exploring "the tension between bodily and social existence, a religious sensibility in a secular world, the inescapable presence of death and loss in daily life." In Philip Roth's *Letting Go*, there is a strangely sweet scene between the constipated husband at work in the bathroom and his wife sitting by the open door, chatting and encouraging his efforts. Laxative abuse features in Ottessa Moshfegh's *Eileen*, a novel driven by a young woman's tortuous struggles with her body.

But what I want to convey here is neither metaphysical nor evidence of some inner drama of repression, emotional withholding, or inability to move on, but a thoroughly prosaic ongoing daily reality. Not *mild*, but severe and chronic, this struggle is brought on by the progressive slowing of the involuntary muscular contractions that move food through our intestines. It is often the first symptom or hint of Parkinson's to appear, as much as a decade before the others more commonly associated with the disease in that pre-diagnosis prodrome phase.

You feel and are bunged up and bloated. Clogged. Blocked. Even if you stop eating, the body continues to produce waste in the form of dead bacteria and discarded cells. If you think about what is piling up inside, you'll end up feeling even more disgusted with yourself. Along with your colon, your mind seems to be in a state of near paralysis. You're preoccupied. Irritable. Irrationally ashamed, fearful of the judgment of others. You develop back pain. Worry that you smell. Soon, you're too uncomfortable and restless to sleep. And of course, it's dangerous. Stools, as doctors call them, can become impacted, block the intestines, cause rupture, a full-on medical emergency—

Let's not go there.

When ordinary remedies fail, you'll naturally enough seek medical advice. Be warned that this may be anticlimactic. Be warned that not all doctors are skilled at dealing with this topic. There is a tendency to relay the same old information, clearly inadequate to the particular situation, in a hyper encouraging jolly tone.

"You did? Really? Oh dear. Still, I do think well worth trying again! If at first, we don't succeed—"

Alternatively, a stern approach, implying that one has cheated or not tried hard enough. "Remember, this must be taken *regularly. Without fail.*"

Add in a reluctance to engage in descriptions of the specifics of how the problem manifests (texture, shape, size, smell, soundscape), of what is *actually happening*, let alone carry out a physical examination. Frustration is inevitable.

Understandable? Yes. Helpful, no.

Even in a population given to the almost compulsive sharing and comparing of medical information as PWP seem to be—and even though it affects our general health, medication absorption, mood, quality of life, i.e., pretty much everything—dealing with all this tends to be a dispiriting, private struggle that most feel is best mentioned only indirectly.

"You okay?"

"Oh, you know. A bit off-colour."

~

When, in 2016, during that innocent time before my diagnosis, I decided to sign up for the trek to Machu Picchu, constipation had been already plaguing me for several years. Travel tended to make it worse. I'd already consulted my doctor several times and had visited a specialist who presented me with a chart indicating the shapes and sizes of stools, from perfect (sausage or snake) to worst. Naturally, I had the worst possible (think rabbit—maybe a large rabbit). I felt there should be more options: fingerling potato, pole bean. No one was able to offer me any conclusive help.

"Could be hormonal," was one half-hearted suggestion. My stools were *obstinate*. My bowels were *lazy*, I'd been told, at which I felt instantly protective, as if a child of mine had been criticized. And I was ready to take down the next person who gave me a lecture on water-drinking, healthy diet, exercise, or described different kinds of laxatives, how they worked, and how I shouldn't overuse them—information I'd been fully aware of for years.

It had got to the point where I was *trying*—or rather deliberately *not* trying, but providing an opportunity for what needed to occur—many times a day, producing no more than a few tiny droppings, and in desperation resorting to a manual method of my own devising.

So how would I manage on a camping trek *at altitude*, which makes constipation worse, with ten or more others sharing the facility: a chemical toilet in a flimsy canvas structure to be erected at each lunch or evening camping spot, the whole increasingly foul sloppy mess to be packed up and carried by a sherpa for the entire trek? I had no idea. But I dearly wanted to go to Peru and walk those ancient trails.

By the fifth day in Cuzco, I'd adjusted well to the thin air, and my chronic problem was no worse than usual. Fluid intake, including the local stimulant and cure-all, coca tea? Prodigious. I actually wept with joy as we set off on the first leg of the trek. I hadn't done more than day-long hikes since my early twenties, and something in me yearned to have nothing to do but put one foot ahead of the other and absorb the land I was passing through, to eat, sleep, and walk some more. It felt hard to justify leaving the rest of the family when it was not for work, but they'd encouraged me. Now I and the six others in the group followed the worn pathway along the dry valley beside the gushing Vilcanota River, snow-peaked mountains to either side, cerulean sky above, prickly pear and other more tree-like cacti dotted in amongst the other unknown-to-me plants and grasses. Later that day, we visited the first set of Inca ruins, then set off for higher ground. Ahead of us were giant hummingbirds, iridescent parrots, queuña and chachacomo trees, orchids, gorgeous Andean cloud forest, enormous views, the ruins of Sayaqmarka, Phuyupatamarka, and Machu Picchu itself, not to speak of thousands of Inca-built steps.

The trek did not disappoint.

The bathroom experience, on the other hand . . . Utterly mortifying. In daylight hours, there was always a lineup to the glorified bucket in its near-transparent shroud. On the way to it, one sherpa would offer a dollop of hand sanitizer and hand out two sheets of whisper-thin paper. Another waited on the way out with soap and a bucket of water for hands. Every sound was audible. (Some people clearly had the opposite problem to mine.) And of course, if one happened to feel "ready" while on the route, the urge had to be ignored, given the area's protected status as a unique environment and World Heritage Site. I'd creep out of my shared tent after dark, marvelling at the southern stars and backwards crescent moon and make my way carefully to the unguarded facility only to emerge luckless, my body fighting itself.

A diet based on white rice was unhelpful. Despite being full of it, I lost ten pounds. But *que sera*, I'd done what I came for. I all but wept again when, hike and goodbye dinner complete, I was shown into my modest B&B accommodation: that white porcelain toilet all mine, in the little shower room.

A colonoscopy is rarely going to be fun, though a dear writer friend was delighted with hers: she stayed awake and journeyed with the camera through the clean, softly undulating folds and found it awe-provoking and beautiful. In contrast, I can claim to have had one of the worst-ever experiences, bar some medical emergency such as a puncture of the intestine. At the time, it was horrific, though now in the telling it veers toward comedy.

It began with two weeks of preparation designed to create the squeaky-clean, camera-ready colon my friend had achieved. The preparation specified a diet guaranteed in my case to make things worse, washed down with laxatives that did not work *at all*, and culminating in a final intensive cleanout involving litres of fluid that I'd heard kept you prisoner in the bathroom for an entire day and brought grown men to tears. Naturally, it had negligible effect on my immobilized system.

I called the health line and was told to relax. Perhaps I was having a delayed reaction. Something would probably happen overnight.

It didn't. Early on the morning of the procedure, I called the clinic to explain how things were. That I had taken everything in the correct order, drunk the litres of fluid, yet been unable to clean myself out *at all*. Come in anyway, said the man I spoke with. Did he not believe me? Think I was avoidant, lazy, or negligent?

At the clinic, I tried again to explain. *Please believe me*, I told the woman with the clipboard. *This is why I am having the procedure.* Well then, we'll see what we can do, she said. A kind nurse took me to a bathroom area, screened but not entirely separate from the waiting area, where others from our small community, some of whom I doubtless pass in the grocery store or town park and who might well recognize me, waited begowned in beds.

Had I had an enema before? Somehow that had been missed. The nurse showed me what to do, tactfully absented herself, returned to inspect the brown, murky result. So it might take more than one, she pronounced. Perhaps three or four. Actually, seven.

By the time my doctor had sent me for this colonoscopy, I'd well and truly lost my sense of smell, another missed Parkinson's indication. (I'd consulted an ENT on that count and been advised I had rhinitis and to rinse my sinuses.) So I could not smell my own shit, but I was of course fully aware that the nurse and those beyond the rather symbolic screens would be unable to avoid the doubtless disgusting odours I was producing. All I could do was apologize—and I did so repeatedly, right up until the moment when they sedated me.

It was rather murky in there still, one of the team reported cheerily when I surfaced, still apologizing. But overall, *reassuring,* the report that followed concluded. Well, good. Great! I'm glad someone's happy.

A sluggish digestive system not only causes its own miseries; it interferes with the absorption of the medication that enables a semi-normal life. Added to that, the more effective laxatives on offer come with a caution that they shouldn't be used for more than a few days in a row, lest you become dependent. Already dependent on so much, I'm prepared to take that risk. However, manufacturers also warn against taking other medications *two hours* either side of them, since those other medications may be poorly absorbed or otherwise negatively impacted. I can't allow that to happen. Added to this, Parkinson's drugs have their own strictures as to when they can be taken in relation to meals. My days are rigidly timetabled, with narrow windows between the dosages when I can eat: a nightmare, or I should more positively say, since when done correctly it can make me feel much better, a *challenge*.

Illness absorbs attention, can narrow our focus, shrink our view, imprison us in our malfunctioning bodies. I try not to let this happen. But some days, my awareness cycles from one problem to another. Can't go. Nausea. Bloating. Gas. Exhaustion. Pain. Tightness. Can't go. Motor symptom breakthrough. Nausea. Bloating. Gas . . . Like interrupted sleep, constipation is one of the invisible, ongoing parts of a complicated tangle of symptoms—one that is in itself horrible but also makes all the rest much worse.

Blah, blah, blah.

Perhaps I am making too much of this? I've always been very sensitive to physical sensations, to the point that my mother used to jokingly call me the Princess and the Pea. Perhaps if I had done better with meditation practice, I'd be more able to detach from discomfort?

Of course, my family cannot but be aware of what's been going on inside me. We used to joke about my gurgling innards and irrepressible farts (now, fingers crossed, less frequent), which they assured me smelled of lavender and roses, but I choose not to update my husband too often about what is going on in my intestines or the associated emotions. "Sorry. A bad day on the bowel front," I might mention to explain lethargy or bad temper, but I gladly spare him the gory details. For obvious reasons, I'd rather he did not associate me with something that potentially produces feelings of disgust.

And there is a silver lining. Since I lack a sense of smell, and therefore don't experience physical revulsion in response to unpleasant odours, I have a new role as the household's go-to person for cleaning up our elderly cat's occasional accidents and dealing with any other foul-smelling substances we encounter at home or abroad. A small thing but cheering. Absolutely. Being useful always feels good.

~

12

How Do I Do This?

The dentist, about to freeze my tooth in preparation for making a crown, pauses, syringe in hand, to ask how I'm doing. I tell him pretty well, considering.

"As for me," he replies, "I've been diagnosed with prostate cancer. Late stage. Not a great prognosis, unfortunately." His assistant pushes aside the light that's beaming down on my face.

"No! I'm so sorry. When did you find out?"

"A couple of weeks ago. So I'm up and down. Well, I know you know what it's like. Makes you *think*— though now with the pain under control, I can at least sleep! And work helps. We'd better get on. Nice and wide, please."

Two newly diagnosed PWP, reeling, have appeared at the support group, together with a woman who has suffered with Parkinson's for thirty years and cannot keep still. When she speaks, everyone seated in the circle of chairs leans forward, frowning as we attempt to decode the sounds she makes.

Our daughter's partner's mother has a diagnosis of multiple myeloma, and our friend Derek is undergoing tests due to a persistent cough. It could've been pneumonia, so we were hoping for that, but it turns out to be cancer. Immunotherapy could help. More tests coming up. It's very worrying, but he seems optimistic and mentions in his message the chance of a visit.

Loss, serious illness, terminal diagnosis, unbearable pain, whether one's own or someone else's—even simple aging—inevitably test a person's philosophy and way of life, if they have one. I am not sure that I do.

Derek stops communicating and his wife, Christine, sets up email updates to his many groups of friends.

She tells us that unfortunately he has the wrong kind of cancer for the immunotherapy. His physical condition is worsening, but much helped by pain relief, and he is back home and enjoying time with his family.

Within what seems like a matter of weeks, he moves to the hospice and we don't get to see him after all.

Christine is a very committed Buddhist, but that isn't something Derek shared. I don't know what his philosophy was, though I sense that it would have been clear-headed, down to earth, free of both illusions and fruitless struggle against the inevitable, and not in any way mystical. On the rational, stoic side of things, perhaps? Before he became a sailor and writer, he studied law. I can picture him wearing a toga and debating ethical, legal, or philosophical points. His questions and examples would be impeccably prepared, his arguments seasoned with irony and articulately expressed.

When we call someone stoical, the implication is that they bear misfortune without too much complaint or being knocked utterly off course. Clearly it is a little more complicated than that. This set of ideas about how to live originated in ancient Greece and was later brought to Rome by Epictetus, an educated, enslaved man who was granted his freedom and went on to establish a school there. He taught that status and wealth do not guarantee freedom and that it is possible to find it even in situations that are fundamentally constraining and restricted: when mortal and seemingly imprisoned in a suffering body, for example. However confined, one still has the ability to choose how to think and react.

The Stoic method is to focus efforts on what we can control: our own responses to situations and events, which should be based on reason, rather than emotion. The path to *eudaimonia*—hard to translate: somewhere between goodness, happiness, and living well—is to learn how to think clearly, see and accept the world as it is, and be guided by reason and a striving toward *aretē* (roughly translated: excellence) with a combination of practical wisdom, justice, moderation, and courage.

Also key to this way of thinking is that all things including riches and status are transitory. Even the memory of glorious deeds, the Stoic emperor Marcus Aurelius (one of Epictetus's pupils) pointed out, is temporary, fading with each year and generation.

These ideas aren't unique to the Stoics. Perhaps it seems counterintuitive, given the earthy, pragmatic tone of Stoic writings and the more subtle and intricate texture of Buddhist thought, but many Stoic recommendations are surprisingly similar to Buddhist ways of thinking. The latter are increasingly popular with contemporary Westerners, including Derek's wife, Christine, and many other of my friends; committed stoics are comparatively rare but do exist. They have their own associations, websites, conferences, and journals.

Buddhism is a religion as well as a philosophy. It comes with new language, concepts, practices, rituals. It's more paradoxical, complicated, subtle, and so seemingly mysterious than Stoicism—and perhaps as a result seems more spiritual and less pragmatic. It is by far the more radical of the two in its insistence that the notion of a stable human "self" is an illusion; there's no such suggestion in Stoic thought.

But both emphasize the importance of seeing reality as it is, free of illusions. Both offer tools or methods to help that process, and both recommend acting in accordance with that reality or natural order, arguing that this will replace a tendency to the frenzied, euphoric, insatiable pursuit of what we call happiness with a calmer, more harmonious state. The two philosophies are in accord as to the helpfulness of living in the present—something I'm increasingly interested in yet find virtually impossible to do. Around 2,400 years ago, Epictetus wrote:

> Remind yourself that you love a mortal, something not your own; it has been given to you for the present, not inseparably nor forever, but like a fig, or a bunch of grapes, at a fixed season of the year, and that if you yearn for it in the winter, you are a fool. If in this way you long for your son, or your friend, at a time when he has not been given to you, rest assured that you are *yearning for a fig in winter*. (Italics mine.)

Death is part of the natural order of things, but how can it be foolish to mourn? We miss our friend, who had been part of our life for two decades.

He and Christine arrived here from Toronto at roughly the same time as we did from London. Derek's book *Godforsaken Sea* had sold so well that it allowed them to leave Toronto and devote themselves to raising their daughter and to pursuing their various interests. Their home was an easy walk from ours, so we were neighbours too. We often met at literary events, shared many New Year's gatherings, read each other's books. Supplied encouragement, gossip, commiseration. We taught a workshop together. My husband and Derek were in the same (all male) book club.

Derek didn't follow suit when Christine immersed herself in Buddhism and meditation and over the years pursued increasingly long silent retreats, but he accepted the changes with interest and humour. (Stoically, you might say.) He wrote, looked out for his elderly mother, fixed up his boat, sailed. He had a voyage planned. Things looked very good.

And then.

Like Stoics, Buddhists cultivate an awareness of the impermanence of all things, including the people we love and care deeply for. Our attachment to them, in particular to their bodies, is seen as a source of suffering. Both traditions recommend contemplation of death and the decay of the body to temper, if not prevent, such attachments. Buddhist instructions for monks to observe and learn from actual or portrayed rotting corpses are striking and graphic—for example, the nine stages of decay beginning with distension and rupture and progressing via exudation and putrefaction to discolouration and desiccation, consumption by animals and birds, dismemberment, reduction to bones, and parching to dust.

Marcus Aurelius reminds readers of his *Meditations* that "the composition of the entire body is subject to putrefaction" and urges them to be aware of death; though a man normally very wary of imagination, he recommends, "When you regard each substance, imagine that it is already being dissolved, is in the midst of transformation, in the process of rotting and being destroyed." Memento mori—reminders of death—feature in Christian traditions, too, often as a warning about the possibility of Hell.

Does impermanence make our attachment to the people and other beings we love any less meaningful? Is imagining the decay of our beloved's body or one's own body a useful preparation for sickness and death? Already sick, I'm willing to consider the idea, but I feel doubtful.

When Andrew Marvell reminded his coy mistress of the long years to come in the tomb and the worms that devour us there, it was a preamble to recommending an approach very different to the Stoic one:

> *Let us roll all our strength and all*
> *Our sweetness up into one ball,*
> *And tear our pleasures with rough strife*
> *Through the iron gates of life:*
> *Thus, though we cannot make our sun*
> *Stand still, yet we will make him run.*

Enjoy the transitory while you can. Let go when you must.

Confronted with his father's approaching death, Dylan Thomas urges him to "rage, rage against the dying of the light," the very opposite of acceptance.

The careful wisdom of ancient philosophies or the poets' white-hot emotional authenticity? Are we allowed *both*? Granted, feelings can be fickle and need to be evaluated, but ignoring them rarely turns out well.

Derek's sudden death invites me to consider how I deal with impermanence and loss. It leads me back to a question that I must (repeatedly) confront with regard to myself: How do I do this? I mean live, of course, not die, though there is that, too, and they do seem to be part of the same thing. At present, I'm still mobile, deeply involved in relationships, engaged in activities that I value. Yet there is that weasel word, *progressive*, which ought to be something good, but actually tells me that my brain rot and multi-symptom situation will inevitably worsen.

I can't find my copy of Viktor Frankl's *Man's Search for Meaning*, which I first read as a teenager and have reread since then, but the library has it, of course. An extraordinary document, about 130 pages long, written over a period of nine days in 1945 by a psychotherapist who had survived several years' incarceration in Nazi concentration camps. It details both the horrific, dehumanizing conditions and the inner life that Frankl believed sustained him (though some luck was also involved). He offers his story as a guide to coping with extreme adversity and avoiding despair.

The core of Frankl's message is that "everything can be taken from a man but one thing: the last of the human freedoms—to choose one's attitude in any given set of circumstances, to choose one's own way." There's a Stoic flavour to this, to be sure, but also a more modern, existentialist slant. The key, he explains, is that a person can make their own meaning, even from terrible experiences. So, for example, could I choose to see my experience with this disease as offering me a perspective that most healthier, normally aging people don't easily access? To call it a gift would be a stretch, but I can say that the experience, while unwelcome, is also an interesting one.

The idea that we have the power to choose what to make of our suffering is bold and inspiring—although I have to say that this time around, I find the words themselves less moving than the physicality of the book itself. They appear on the sixty-sixth page of the Beacon Press edition and its corner has been turned down repeatedly, and likewise the corners of the four pages that follow it, in which he considers situations such as sickness and imminent death.

But is this personal transcendence of horror truly possible? Psychiatrist Thomas Szasz (*The Myth of Mental Illness*) is not alone in having criticized Frankl's assertions and attitudes. Some have even doubted parts of his story. But eighty years after the words were written, many still seek them out, turn and return to them, find something of worth, copy them into a notebook, take a screenshot, bend over the corner of the page.

In *Intoxicated by My Illness*, Anatole Broyard offers another form of radical acceptance. "Every seriously ill person needs to develop a style for his illness," Broyard asserts. "Only by insisting on your style can you keep from falling out of love with yourself as the illness attempts to diminish or disfigure you. Sometimes your vanity is the only thing that's keeping you alive." Style? Vanity extolled as motivation? Part of me pulls away from the intense narcissism he apparently extols, yet why not? Broyard wished to use his disease to become a more intense version of who he had been. Not for him the "no-self." He wanted *more* self. He wanted to win. On paper, he does. Broyard, it strikes me, is Viktor Frankl in a sharp suit.

One afternoon in September, we gather on a sun-drenched hillside to remember Derek. It has scarcely rained since June; the heat is intense and dry, the sky an acute and brilliant blue. Some—those who thought to wear broad-brimmed hats—sit in rows facing a low improvised stage. Others stand close to the house in a shrinking stripe of shade, and a few sit on what, before the drought, used to be a grassy bank. Nigel, the man with the red-light hat from the Parkinson's support group, is here with his wife, along with writers, adventurers, sailors, farmers, neighbours . . . We've eaten, drunk, hugged, laughed, mingled, wept, gazed at the displays of photographs and books. Wasps cluster around the remaining food; above it all, perpetually hungry swallows dive and reel.

The last notes of an Irish ballad fade to nothing. We hear tell of our friend's deeds and sayings, his qualities. Kindness. Wry humour. Intelligence. Sense of justice. Tolerance, except of those who abuse others. Rationality. Curiosity, appetite for adventure. Courage. Steadfastness. The use of the past tense is still a shock.

Richard and I reach for each other's hands when Christine steps forward and stands in the sun looking out at us all. There's a silence before she thanks us for being there and then addresses us without looking at her notes. Her voice vibrates with all she feels and has come to understand as she describes her husband and their life together, their joint ventures and adventures, and also how they had lived this last unwelcome part of their time together, during which they managed each in their own way to not merely accept but embrace the experience and find a way to make it theirs—to fill the last weeks with love and grow yet closer than before. She touches her chest, just to the left, as she speaks.

She is both happy and sad. Grateful. Gentle yet also incandescent. Somehow, she has remained emotionally open and at the same time dealt with the demanding practicalities of sickness and death, sustained herself, accepted help as needed, kept in touch

with all Derek's friends. How very well she has han-
dled what's been dealt to them. It seems to me that
she has, they both have, done this hard thing as well
as it can possibly be done. They have committed to
what they did not wish for and lived it to the full.

I hope to do the same.

13

~

In Person

On a bright day about two years after I first knew I needed a neurologist, I have my first in-person consultation.

It's a familiar set-up: a low-rise block attached to a small, dreary shopping mall surrounded by parking areas decorated with the usual dusty, drought-tolerant bushes. A pharmacy on ground level. Optometrist nearby. An elevator with a long list of doctor names beside it—he's on the top floor. A stifling utilitarian corridor of office doors. Off screen, in real life, it's a shock. *He's enormous!* I realize as I stand to follow him into the consulting room. Six foot six and proportionally built. A giant! Not so exotic as the dream cyclops or Phyllis with one leg, but certainly at odds with the proportions of the doors. Added to that is a certain fishbowl effect from being in a corner room with large windows on two sides.

"Well, how are you?" he asks. I tell him how I have struggled with implementing his recent advice to increase the frequency of my medication, and that I think this is because to do so will mean acknowledging that my condition is, far too soon for my liking, *progressing*. He nods. On the practical front, I point out that when the intervals between doses are shorter, everything will become more inconvenient and anti-social in terms of mealtimes and social activities.

"Good point. Of course, I'm not going to order you to make the change. It's a trade-off. You'll do it when it seems worthwhile to you. When you do so, I recommend you give it a proper trial."

He watches me walk. Stands gigantically behind me and pulls my shoulders sharply backwards. Asks me to touch my nose with my fingertip. Draw a circle. Count backwards while doing various things with my hands.

"I really wouldn't know you had it," he says. I'm at the peak of a dose; we both know things could be different a few hours later. He manages to end every session, virtual, phone, or in person, on some kind of positive note. This is probably why I feel better after seeing him. The disease, not the doctor, is the problem.

14

~

Downsized

So it's just sooner than we thought. Somewhat more urgent.

I know you're right. But really, must we? Because here, our children played in the snow, brought their friends, slept with their first loves, wept over breakups (also, there was that party that got out of hand), and bit by bit became able to leave. Because families of deer also live here, walk out of the woods, graze, twitch their ears at our small domestic sounds, rest in the sun, sometimes peer through the windows of the house we built. Eagles cruise overhead, settle on snags, make their strange, fluting cry. Waxwings feast on our berries. Vegetables root, sprout, fruit, ripen, rot. Let's not forget the oh-so-prolific plum tree. All the other fruit trees! Mere whips when we planted them. And there's the layered, paper-thin, pistachio-green bark of the arbutus: how it darkens in stages to a glowing chestnut brown. The crack and rustle as it splits and peels. Here stands my writing cabin that our neighbours put up for us, and inside it the curvy worktable and bookcase you made to fit the space. Our rainwater collection system. The trail at the back. The sun-drenched valley beyond the trees. The sky! That scrap of ocean view beyond which on very clear days a distant mountain hangs like a mirage.

Can we not stay and let the garden do its own thing, the deer fences collapse? Allow gutters to block, paint to peel, wood to crack and rot, mushrooms to sprout? Dine on them and berries, apples, and plums, potatoes, volunteer squash. Stop paying bills; use the tank of collected rainwater, add a composting toilet. If it came to it, we could live in just part of the house, wrapped in blankets half the year, and eventually be left out in the woods for the vultures, eagles, and the cougar said to live nearby. Extreme, I admit. But why not wait a few more years and make the move only when being here becomes intolerable or dangerous, and then move directly to a fully accessible condo in the city? If, that is, I—

Sorry!

We'll not go there. And no, of course not. Yes, better now than to wait until we're utterly overwhelmed and unable. No, I certainly don't want you walking on the roof again! And you, thankfully, don't want to. Nor do you want to stain the siding, clean out rainwater collection filters and tank, mend the broken irrigation pump, deal with another massive wind-felled tree . . . For my part, I can neither regulate the vigour of the garden vegetation nor bear to see it strangled by brambles and broom.

Agreed: neither of us want to lavish our remaining energy and my relatively good years in an ongoing battle to maintain our home. Add in the cost of heating a space designed for at least four . . .

We're sitting opposite each other at the big cherry and maple table you made. It's a matter of imagining ourselves differently, you say. We can adapt, you tell me. We came here. We're good at this, you say, reaching across and taking my hand in yours as you do so, and what more could I ask?

~

We jettison the possibly useful stuff that's been allowed to lurk and reproduce itself for years in the garage, heave bags of unloved clothes to the thrift store. Books. Will you read it again? Does it have sentimental value? We discard a good third of our library, selling and giving away what we can. And you sell or give away your planer, saws, sander, and benches from the workshop. In the last few weeks, we take down pictures and photographs, decide which to keep. Wrap pans and dishes. Pack, tape, label.

The movers (a family of fundamentalist Christians) rattle up at eight in the monring in the very same van that was overdue for retirement seventeen years ago when they moved us in. We spend an entire day (and fifteen hundred dollars) on the actual transition. It's lonely. You're in the new place directing the placement of each load; I'm in the old one, cleaning behind two middle-aged men and a boy as they cheerfully empty our rooms, eschewing breaks and making conscientious little piles of any small change they find as they go. As we work, the sounds we all make gradually gain a strange dryness and sharpness, the beginning of an echo.

Ten hours pass before the van coughs into life for the last load, lumbers down the first part of the steep driveway (remember: an ice sheet in winter, not to be missed). It vanishes into the shadows, squeals through the narrow part between the stand of old cedars. Finally, a roar as it struggles up the short uphill section and out onto the road (a nasty turn, also not to be missed).

And now there's only the wind in the trees; indoors, my own over-loud footsteps as I walk slowly around a strange, beautiful but empty version of the place we built, lived and loved in, which belongs now to someone new and from which we must somehow detach ourselves.

~

Our new place has the right number of rooms, including the possibility of a downstairs mini-suite should stairs one day become impossible. It has good light, a spacious kitchen. Room for a workspace each. With ingenuity, there's just enough space for a guest or two. We can work, eat, sleep, wash, socialize. There are some pleasing aesthetic touches. Solar panels to shrink the hydro bill. A good park just steps away. Walking distance from the library and shops.

There's a shortage of such places, as there is of other affordable accommodation, the sort needed for young families, for front-line workers, students, and those with serious mental health or disability challenges. Some people sleep in the parks and vans nearby. I know we're lucky. Very lucky. Yet for months, I mourn what used to be and notice only faults. A yard overplanted with mechanical repetitions of the same four unlovable shrubs, situated often in defiance of the light, soil, and water requirements of said plants, many of which look stunted and sick. A huge area of make-work *lawn*, of all things. And the soundscape! Glugging ravens have been replaced by quarrelling crows, and just as we'd anticipated, there's much more human and traffic noise. Nasty fake wood-grain flooring in the bathrooms. Poor-quality siding beginning to cup and buckle. A long concrete path that slicks and freezes in winter.

"How do you like your new home?" we're asked, naturally enough. Some ask more than once. Some even dare to ask, "Are you *loving* your new home?" I won't pretend but try to adopt a reasonable, neutral tone as I explain that well, I did of course much prefer the other, though it was increasingly impractical, and this has its plus points.

Inside, I burn with outrage, fury . . . I can only think of one plus point: it's *convenient*. Not a fair exchange for *wonderful*. An expulsion from our Eden, this oh-so-sensible move stands for the whole of being sick. I remind myself it was voluntary and is irrevocable. That as Epictetus said, it is folly to yearn for a fig in winter. Order that same self not to sulk! To get on with it because here is where we are and so it goes, until—

Barefoot, silent, I enter the cool tiled corridor that leads to the small utility area. I've come to fetch the washing to hang outside. Ahead of me, another door bars the way to the soundproofed workspace that you installed for your singing and guitar playing in what may ultimately end up as a disability suite. Heavy padded drapes, thick carpet, and black egg-box-like foam cover windows, floor, walls. It's very effective. You're protected from outside sounds, liberated from distracting self-consciousness or concern about disturbing others. Just occasionally, when you sing and strum at your very loudest, faint sounds emerge, as if from a distant radio to nearby rooms, but no one mentions this to you.

The inner door is closed, meaning do not disturb. I can hear some muted strumming on the guitar. Even so, soundproofing works both ways. I know I can ever so gently open the washing machine door and ease out our clothes and sheets. I'm reaching forward, my hand almost on the door when you, perhaps three metres away from me, start to sing. Your voice is distanced, even though we are so close, yet it doesn't matter at all, nor that I catch only some of the words. What is this?

I stand, not just ears but every cell of me open to absorb the flow of notes, this sung music you are making, every note. Your voice and the song itself, tender, strong, angry, suffering, bitter, transcendent, intimate, perfectly express who you are and the fact of it happening at last.

How fortunate I am to stand here, transfixed, at noon in the cool dusk of our windowless utility room, wet-faced and uninvited.

It's not just the beauty of the music that slays me. It's the fulfillment of the work that has gone into it, the commitment. How you blended persistence and postponement, delayed, lapsed, sang in the shower and the woods, studied the music you love, scrawled ideas in notebooks. And *kept* them.

I confess of course, and as hoped, you don't mind at all.

It's not long now until you'll emerge from the studio and sing with me present in the shared broad daylight of the living room. Shy after so much private rehearsal, it's hard to keep your eyes open and to bring what has been private into a shared space. It's the same for many writers. I know you'll be able to do it. Next step is a *solo debut* (the words make us laugh, but that's what it is): a performance at the local Legion's open mic, eyes almost always open, to an evening audience that includes friends, our son, total strangers, and no small number of other musicians. There's eating, drinking, a girls' night out—but there is also your voice, a little tight to begin with, fuller and easier with each song as you lose the nerves and move from the covers to your own songs. I lean across and ask our son, Jimmy, right in his ear, "Do you have face-ache too?" Our grins grow wider still.

To come: all-day band rehearsals. Tortuous discussion over the band's name: Mercy Dogs. A real stage, raising you all above the crowd. Decent sound. Lighting, projection. Soon I'll see you stand right at the front of that stage in your loose silver pinstriped suit, gladly meeting the collective gaze of the audience, ready to go. *1-2-3-*, a gasp of breath, and all at once a hall full of sound—bold, fast, angry, loud. Patrick bossing with the drums. Guitar and bass cross back and forth, and your voice, tonight 100 percent full-on astounding, holds, rises out of all this sound, and leads the song where it needs to go.

I'll be dancing with our poet friend Shirley and the couple who now live in our previous house. Your poor sister, ear-plugged, recovering from a concussion, slapping her hand on her thigh. Wonderful! But I treasure those moments in the utility room even more.

Deferred desires often shrivel into mere fantasies. I have feared at times that you would not get this far. That you might have left it too late. I have worried that it was a sad flaw in our life together, a lack of balance or fairness, since after all, I've been able to fulfill my calling. I have doubly cursed my disease for making me unable to pull my weight, and I've feared that my increasing needs for help would develop to a point where they impeded you just as you began. Not so. Didn't happen. Is it possible that my illness, despite its destructive nature, might accidentally have created a useful sense of urgency, pushed things along?

A nice thought.

In any case, since the day I crept into the utility room and overheard your voice, I have forgiven this house. I've started to see not what it lacks and instead to love it for what it has allowed. For the way your voice lives more openly with us—a fascinating creature, demanding, sometimes capricious, certainly not any kind of pet. For the way we two now live together, part-time writer and musician, chatting about progress or its opposite at the end of the day, each encouraging the other. This is something I've not experienced before and did not anticipate.

Outside, it's not the other house and never will be. But the sickly rhododendrons are long gone. We're growing garlic, lettuce, tomatoes, extra basil for our daughter. Washing flaps on the line in the backyard. We sometimes hear owls at night, and we plan, when the fall comes, to sow wildflowers to replace most of the lawn.

15

~

A Curious Tale

Patrick drops by at the hottest point of a hot August afternoon. He's texted to check we're around, so we meet him at the gate. A big man, flushed, damp, glistening, he insists, still catching his breath, that he's enjoyed the walk, part of a recent resolve to take more exercise. An accomplished visual artist and musician, Pat knows a huge assortment of people and has worked in many different capacities. In the way that some visitors arrive with a bunch of garden flowers or a bag of cookies, Pat tends to begin a visit with some kind of information or news.

"I saw such an interesting thing on the way—" He pauses momentarily, looks from one to the other of us to ensure we're paying attention. "At the top of the hill near the hydro station. You know the spot where there's a bit of a pull-over on the other side of the road and people sometimes park in summer to sell fruit or spot prawns or whatever? You know where I mean?" Again, the pause. We blink, nod. "I'd just come around that curve, and I see a woman standing right there wearing just bikini bottoms. No top. And suddenly I'm very curious—"

I can't hear *curious* without thinking of *Alice's Adventures in Wonderland,* a book I've loved ever since my sister first read it to me—the wild story, Tenniel's illustrations, but most of all the girl herself, that plucky, questioning child in her knee-length petticoat and frock. Persistent and resilient, the perfect protagonist and a powerful antidote to Victorian tendencies to view children as either romantically pure and close to nature or inherently evil until the devil could be beaten out of them.

"Burning with curiosity" is how Carroll describes Alice in the third paragraph of *Wonderland,* when she impulsively follows the white rabbit down its hole and finds herself sliding, then falling. And of course, Carroll's story was written at a time when curiosity, especially female curiosity, was still of dubious value and often construed as an impertinence that led to catastrophe, grief, and an overheated brain.

"I didn't see much," Patrick elaborates, "because I didn't want to stop and gawp, and as I came round the bend, I realized she was holding a sign that read 'Stop Bullying!' at chest level. You could only see her breasts from a certain angle, and once the road curved, you saw only the sign, blotting out her chest. So, I'm wondering, Can people in the cars even see that she is topless? I'm assuming she wants them to? But maybe not? And then does she mean any specific bullying? Is this serious, or a joke that I'm not getting? What's going on?" Neither of us responds, and the vacuum following his question fills with the collective hum of the bees performing their complicated dance in the lavender bushes to either side of the path to the cooler indoors.

Two centuries before *Alice* was published in 1865, Charles Perrault, a French collector of fairy tales, offered the following as a moral lesson arising from the story of Bluebeard: "Curiosity, in spite of its appeal, often leads to deep regret. To the displeasure of many a maiden, its enjoyment is short lived. Once satisfied, it ceases to exist, and always costs dearly." I do of course disagree with the gender bias and absolutism.

Like Alice, the young wife in Perrault's version of Bluebeard is very curious, to the point that she abandons her guests and nearly falls down the stairs in her eagerness to reach the secret door and turn the forbidden key in the lock. Her eagerness has been stoked by her husband's repeated warning not to enter that room and by her suspicion that, since no one seems to know what happened to his previous wives, he may well have something to hide. Their mutilated bodies lie, of course, just to the other side of that door in what Angela Carter calls "the bloody chamber."

Alice's adventures, however, culminate in a farcical trial scene during which she is moved to contradict the King's and Queen's judgments, then quarrels with them so vehemently over the illogical procedures of

the court that she is expelled—or expels herself—
from Wonderland and wakes in a meadow with her
head in her sister's lap. The fate of Bluebeard's wife
depends on which version you read. Some versions
show her duly punished as promised, warning the
reader against disobedience. Perrault, however, allows
her to be saved from her murderous husband by her
brother's sword.

We're still on the path, standing in full sun.

"So, is she against the bullying of women who are
or want to be topless? Or all bullying in general?"
Patrick wipes sweat from his face with the back of
one hand, continues: "And again, how—just how is
this protest supposed to work? What would be the
measure of success? How long is she going to stand
there? And then I saw there was a guy, too, a skinny,
stubbly-looking guy—"

"Also in swimwear?" I ask, mock-solemn.

"No," Patrick says, sighing regretfully as he shuts
down an entire and attractive range of enquiry. The
man accompanying the topless woman was neither
naked nor sporting a Speedo. He wore jeans and a
white T-shirt and stood a few feet away from the topless woman pointing vigorously, over and over, "like a
kind of living GIF. 'Look! Look! She's topless! Stop bullying!' What the hell or on earth are they trying to do?"

It used to be commonplace to talk negatively of *idle*
curiosity, meaning interest that has no justification,

purpose, or profitable outcome, which might distract the person concerned (especially when female) from doing whatever servile task they were supposed to be doing.

Contemporary scientists identify three or more types of curiosity: diversive, epistemic, and empathic. Idle would likely be categorized as diversive: playful, free-ranging, omnidirectional, and, I would add, very enjoyable as well as useful if there is something you need to distract yourself from.

According to a 2010 study, curiosity may bring us pleasure or pain, depending on whether we are in an open, free-flowing, unattached way interested in the missing information (diversive, pleasant) or, at the other end of the spectrum, desperately and urgently needing it (epistemic, painful).

Bluebeard's wife is seeking vital information, so that would be a case of the epistemic kind. I think Alice engages in all three sorts, but right now I'm most interested in the diversive kind.

I'm convinced that diversive curiosity can be therapeutic. Alice wonders. She asks herself questions that she cannot answer. How will she relate to her feet now that her head is so much farther away from them? What might the flame of a candle look like when it is blown out? She questions the inhabitants of the potentially terrifying world she finds herself in as to how and why things occur as they do, what they mean. She persists even when the answers she receives are ridiculous or incomprehensible.

The simple act of posing these questions creates for Alice a distance from the hallucinatory parade of bizarre characters and events she encounters, and this slight detachment allows her to avoid terror, bewilderment, and sheer overload while her body grows and shrinks and she attempts to hold logical conversations with the likes of the Mad Hatter and a madder still Queen of Hearts.

Curiosity is for adults too. Like Alice, I've fallen into a hole. Very deep. More like a mine shaft. No white rabbit. I just fell and ended up in another rather hostile place with a Parkinson's diagnosis and a lot of people in a similar predicament. There's certainly ample potential for terror, yet it does help to try, even if I fail, to understand the mechanisms of the disease and what I can do to help myself, and it very much helps to be curious about other people who've experienced the same fall and about how they think and feel. Who were they before all this? What might I learn from them? Why us? How come we are all here? Is it our fault? What can we do? How can we help each other? What *is* this thing?

Curiosity allows me to feel less trapped, to distract and entertain myself. It helps me to explore in manageable pieces matters that otherwise might paralyze me. And by asserting that some aspects of any situation—even this one, its trajectory so clearly down and rather fast at that—are unknown, curiosity fosters hope. It creates a space for possibility, for surprise.

Curiosity can make us happier. And it's free.

Though there are limits.

When it comes to medical specifics, questions about cause and cure shift gear into something more intense, a need for knowledge driven by an unrequited yearning for an escape from the current predicament. For answers, solutions, resolution. I'm passionately interested in the problem this disease presents—yet poorly qualified to investigate, contribute, or even confidently evaluate much of what knowledge exists. I can and will learn but must ultimately rely on scientists to deploy professional (epistemic) curiosity along with analysis and other skills as they investigate the questions that may, via yet further proliferating questions, eventually lead to understanding and cure.

I'm dependent, in other words. At most, my role, my contribution might be as a participant in a double-blind trial or an activist raising awareness and funds. I'm necessarily a spectator cheering others on—struggling to decode the ever-proliferating studies and evaluate the most fruitful, trying to make a palatable, curiosity-based cocktail from far too many supplementary ingredients: hope, awe, impatience, disappointment, gratitude.

Science is slow; life is short.

I would say to Charles Perrault that it's not so simple. I'd say curiosity does frequently make us happier, but yes, I do grant that it can sometimes—whatever our gender—have unexpected consequences and take us where we do not wish to go.

~

Not long ago, after a quick plunge into some need-to-know medical reading, I slid into initially pleasant speculation about the eponymous naming of diseases: Crohn, Alzheimer, Huntington, Hodgkin . . . and another, closer to home. How much of an honour can it really be, I wondered, to be forever remembered for one's connection to a life-ruining set of symptoms? How does that happen? Does the scientific community consult the person concerned? No, I soon and very easily learned.

And then I still more or less idly wondered, What kind of man was James Parkinson? It was easy to find out, and the answer seems initially so heart-warmingly benign: a kind and sought-after doctor who lived from 1775 to 1824, a lifelong political activist concerned with bringing about universal suffrage. Extraordinary for his era. A lovely man! Also a prolific writer, which further inclines me to like him. His published works include *Hints for the Improvement of Trusses*, "intended to render their use less inconvenient, and to prevent the necessity of an understrap . . . for the use by the labouring poor"; *Dangerous Sports: A Tale Addressed to Children*; *Organic Remains of a Former World* (a paleontological study of fossil discoveries in three volumes, containing Parkinson's illustrations as well as text); and *Some Account on the Effects of Lightning.*

This was all such fun!

And what exactly did the good doctor do to be forever cursed by association with a disease already well-known in ancient Greece, China, and India and now inflicting itself on ten million people worldwide, of whom I am one? Again, the answer came all but instantly: he wrote and published in 1817 *An Essay on the Shaking Palsy*. It's freely available in the public domain.

At this point, just moments away from crossing the threshold into what soon became a version of Carter's bloody chamber, I could have paused, evaluated, and refrained from moving forward without some mental equivalent of protective clothing, but, curious, curious, oh so curious, I plunged right in.

The essay's first few passages were harmless, rather quaint. And then came the word *hitherto* . . . I knew that after *hitherto* a shift of gears was inevitable, yet curious, gripped, I read on.

Hitherto the patient will have experienced but little inconvenience; and befriended by the strong influence of habitual endurance, would perhaps seldom think of his being the subject of disease, except when reminded of it by the unsteadiness of his hand, whilst writing or employing himself in any nicer kind of manipulation. But as the disease proceeds, similar employments are accomplished with considerable difficulty, the hand failing to answer with exactness to the dictates of the will. Walking becomes a task which cannot be performed without considerable attention. The legs are not raised to that height, or with that promptitude which the will directs, so that the utmost care is necessary to prevent frequent falls.

At this period the patient experiences much inconvenience, which unhappily is found daily to increase. The submission of the limbs to the directions of the will can hardly ever be obtained in the performance of the most ordinary offices of life. The fingers cannot be disposed of in the proposed directions and applied with certainty to any proposed point. As time and the disease proceed, difficulties increase: writing can now be hardly at all accomplished; and reading, from the tremulous motion, is accomplished with some difficulty. Whilst at meals the fork not being duly directed frequently fails to raise the morsel from the plate: which, when seized, is with much difficulty conveyed to the mouth. At this period the patient seldom experiences a suspension of the agitation of his limbs. Commencing, for instance in one arm, the wearisome agitation is borne until beyond sufferance, when by suddenly changing the posture it is for a time stopped in that limb, to commence, generally, in less than a minute in one of the legs, or in the arm of the other side. Harassed by this tormenting round . . .

~

"I wondered," Patrick says, "whether to cross over and very politely just ask, find out what they were trying to convey. But there was traffic. Very respect-ful. No one was honking. But she might have felt I was encroaching on her. He might have got aggres-sive. Or, who knows, wanted a fight!" He looks again from one to the other of us. Sighs. Folds his arms across his chest. "Now," he says, "I wish I had taken the risk. I can't stop thinking about it. Why did she choose to expose herself, especially since holding the sign rather negated the gesture?" Pat's being so curi-ous is one of the reasons we like him so much. And not just curious but *idly* so.

"You say choose, but did she choose?" Richard asks. It seems like a big question, and at last we decide to move discussion of the Very Curious Affair of the Topless Bullying Protest to the much cooler indoors.

The propensity to lean forward becomes invincible, and the patient is thereby forced to step on the toes and fore part of the feet, whilst the upper part of the body is thrown so far forward as to render it difficult to avoid falling on the face . . . at the same time, irresistibly impelled to take much quicker and shorter steps, and thereby to adopt unwillingly a running pace. In some cases, it is found necessary entirely to substitute running for walking; since otherwise the patient, on proceeding only a very few paces, would inevitably fall.

"So, the stubbly man," Richard says as I spoon ice into three big tumblers, add sprigs of homegrown mint. "Maybe he's the bully, and he bullied her into it?" I fetch the big jug from the fridge, pour.

"You think he threatened her?" Patrick asks.

"Well, it's possible," Richard says.

"Why does the topless woman have to be a victim?" I ask. "And why would stubbly, himself a bully, bully her into an anti-bullying protest?"

"If that is what this is," adds Patrick.

"Doesn't make sense!" I tell them.

The power of conveying the food to the mouth is at length so much impeded that he is obliged to consent to be fed by others. The bowels, which had been all along torpid, now, in most cases, demand stimulating medicines of very considerable power: the expulsion of the faeces from the rectum sometimes requiring mechanical aid. As the disease proceeds towards its last stage, the trunk is almost permanently bowed, the muscular power is more decidedly diminished, and the tremulous agitation becomes violent. The patient walks now with great difficulty ... His words are now scarcely intelligible; and he is not only no longer able to feed himself, but when the food is conveyed to the mouth, so much are the actions of the muscles of the tongue, pharynx, &c. impeded by impaired action and perpetual agitation, that the food is with difficulty retained in the month until masticated; and then as difficultly swallowed. Now also, from the same cause, another very unpleasant circumstance occurs—

"Maybe it's the other way around," I suggest. "Maybe *she* made *Stubbly* do it. Maybe it's a punishment!"

"What for, *bullying*?"

"Or—suppose they are playing some adult version of Truth or Dare? They've been given this to do; she's up for it, but he's reluctant, and— No, wait! Could they not both be part of an experimental improv theatre company visiting the island for just one day? Theme, costumes, and both their character names were drawn out of a hat this morning. Then they took it from there. Suppose what Pat saw was just a fragment of this extended improvisation that began at dawn and will end at dusk. This is their actual job! The arts council funds them to do it. What do you think?"

As the debility increases and the influence of
the will over the muscles fades away, the tremulous agitation becomes more vehement. It
now seldom leaves him for a moment; but
even when exhausted nature seizes a small
portion of sleep, the motion becomes so violent as not only to shake the bed-hangings,
but even the floor and sashes of the room. The
chin is now almost immovably bent down
upon the sternum. The slops with which he is
attempted to be fed, with the saliva, are continually trickling from the mouth. The power
of articulation is lost. The urine and faeces are
passed involuntarily; and at the last, constant
sleepiness, with slight delirium, and other
marks of extreme exhaustion, announce the
wished-for release.

An Essay on the Shaking Palsy is seventy-two pages
long. In subsequent sections, Parkinson presents case
studies and describes an autopsy. Later he speculates,
wrongly, as to causes. It is a horrific read, especially
for one of the afflicted or someone close to them, yet,
one can argue, appropriately so. It's certainly one that
I brought upon myself. And despite his lurid prose
style and the shock it has delivered, I feel that the
author's intentions were good. He wanted to convey a
ghastly reality and to provoke sympathy and interest,
not the awkward, nervous mirth the sheer vividness
of his description provokes in some modern readers

used to a cooler scientific tone. Despite the shock of being plunged into the living hell Parkinson saw, I'll admit to liking the man for looking so keenly at the world about him, for the way he felt it was important to do that and to describe what he saw. That, surely, must be the beginning of being curious about and then developing a greater understanding of anything, and from there to eventually improving upon the status quo.

Parkinson's scientific curiosity, compassionate but not personally needy—*epistemic*, perhaps—made it possible for others to be aware of and curious about the condition he so vividly described, to seek to understand its possible causes and discover treatments. Innumerable studies, speculations, and a hundred and fifty years later, the essay bore tangible fruit in 1967 when levodopa was first successfully used to alleviate symptoms.

In the following five decades, in increasingly sophisticated laboratories teams of scientists able to draw on a huge bank of knowledge, derived from the array of scientific, medical, and technical discoveries made since Parkinson wrote, have continued the project he began. There have been no definitive breakthroughs. Knowledge accumulates and complicates. One question often leads to another, without seeming to bring us closer to the useful answer, to the closure we crave. Cause and cure remain elusive.

The world we inhabit, altogether more complex than Parkinson's, is one in which money speaks volumes and the desire for profit is an inevitable part of the story. Every year, hundreds of millions of dollars are spent worldwide on Parkinson's research. Investors want return. Some enquiries attract more funding than others. Repurposing an existing already-patented drug, for example, will, however promising it seems, ultimately generate much less revenue than finding and patenting a new one, so may proceed slowly, if at all.

We hold our noses, donate. Charitable foundations and community groups add their hard-earned fundraised dollars to government and corporate investment. Meanwhile, the number of cases in the US alone grows by an estimated ninety thousand a year. Dealing with the good doctor's disease costs that same country an estimated fifty billion dollars a year.

And it's not only the bills to be paid and the number of people suffering that continually expand, but likewise the list of symptoms. Some say there are forty or more. The *Essay* documented just a handful: tremor (a symptom not experienced by about a third of us), shuffling gait, shrunken handwriting, extreme constipation, weakness, drooling, loss of the ability to eat and speak. Now we have dystonia: excruciating clenching of muscles and tendons, often in the feet. Freezing: both feet may suddenly seem bonded to the floor as if by powerful magnets. You simply cannot lift them, must stand there, perhaps in a crowded supermarket, street, or subway station, perhaps alone in your own home, desperate to reach the bathroom where more problems wait for you, yet unable to lift a foot or walk until you or someone else can find a way to distract your brain, to break the spell. Throw in what is politely termed cognitive decline. And add in masking, in some ways one of the worst, also very common: your facial muscles become rigid, increasingly reluctant to smile or frown, to move at all, so that you barely signal emotions of any kind (and then realize you are not feeling them either). Your face is a lump of seemingly lifeless flesh from which peer out a pair of angry, lost, terrified eyes that scarcely resemble those you remember you once had; one of your friends passes in the street without at first recognizing you.

And oh, the little things—your stupid brain is also neglecting to make your eyelids blink; those alarming new eyes are first dry and itchy and then watering profusely; and meanwhile your scalp is drenched with oil, and no one can explain why—it's enough to drive you insane—and probably will, since dementia is very likely indeed—

Stop. Stop. Stop.

Confronted with this threat, Bluebeard's wife would use delaying tactics and count on her rescue by others. (This is what we PWP mainly do.) But what about Alice? Would Carroll create, and Tenniel illustrate, Alice's encounter with a brave and dogged Parkinson's-afflicted character as a kind of alternative to old Father William or one of the mad queens?

What would an elderly Alice, herself afflicted, do and say? Insist that her malfunctioning brain (portrayed by Tenniel as floating mid-air, continually vanishing and reappearing, rather like the Cheshire Cat) stop behaving so badly and explain itself? Insist on better service? Order it to pull up its socks and be presented in return with baffling nonsensical riddles of her brain's (and is it or is it not then *her own*) making? Throw a tantrum, tell it she knows it is a hallucination, and at the end of a count of ten wake up back in the meadow, leaving the stupid organ at the bottom of the mine shaft? Realize as she begins the count to ten that it is actually impossible; there will be no return to the surface.

~

"We need more information," Pat says. "I'm going back there right now. Thanks for the tea!" He stands and quickly checks the table for anything he might have left. Thanking him in turn for his curious tale, we accompany him to the door, then watch him jog down the lavender-lined path, out the gate and on to the trail: no longer idly curious, but a man who needs to know.

16

~

Mary-Ann

There is a part of me, sometimes quite a large part, that longs for my mother, or *a* mother, or anyone with a kind voice and skin smelling faintly of Nivea cream to wrap me in their arms and say that everything will be all right. Stroke my forehead and wipe it with a damp washcloth. Close the curtains against the glaring sunlight and put that little brass bell on my bedside table so I can ring if I need more lemon barley water or feel like I might throw up. And later as I begin to recover, to bring me a small, special meal decorated with a garden flower, a colouring book beside it on the tray . . . It's unlikely, though, since my mother has been dead for almost a decade. And I am very glad that I've not had to tell her about my diagnosis.

"Oh?" says my New Zealand sister, Jan. "Because?"

No mother wants to hear such news, and no daughter wants to inflict it; if this diagnosis fell to one of my own children, I would yearn for some god to bargain with, beg to endure it myself instead. And just like any mother, ours would have been aghast. But then, tending to be skeptical concerning doctors (she so rarely had need of or encountered one herself) and scientists (impossible to understand), she'd defend herself by not believing it. Did I get a second opinion? And then she would question me as to the symptoms, at first making small noises in her throat, then silent as the list progressed. Then—

"It would have to be *someone's fault*." I hear my words echo faintly back to me as I speak.

"The fault of someone not her. Yours! Of course," Jan says. "Disease well-timed on your part. Congratulations."

I wouldn't have told Mum until I absolutely had to.

~

She never seemed even slightly unwell. Viruses shrivelled at the first encounter with her immune system, as did sales assistants or waiters if she had a complaint. Everything about her was wholesome and naturally strong. She slept soundly, ate well, never needed to even take over-the-counter medication. She walked a lot. She was vigorous and energetic in everything she undertook to the point that when she left a room, conversation withered and all but died until she returned. As for vices, she drank only champagne, which appeared a few times a year for birthdays or my parents' anniversary. She even managed to smoke in an exemplary, almost healthy way: at the most, one mild, filtered cigarette a day, after dinner, taken in her favourite armchair with her feet up. This was a relaxing, healthy thing to do, and she absolutely was not, was *not, addicted.*

Mum often brought her good health into conversation. Doctor's comments on the excellence of her various bodily systems were quoted. Her teeth, too, were famously strong, cavity free. This, she told us, was due to our grandmother giving her ham bones to gnaw on when she was teething.

Provided they were not too close to home, she liked to hear the horrible details of sickness and disability. How brightly their ordeals made her good fortune shine in contrast! She was also drawn to speculation as to what levels of loss and dysfunction were bearable, and at what point *life would not be worth living.* She set the bar high: loss of independence, such as needing help with bodily functions, or reduced mobility seemed to her a clear threshold not to be crossed. As she grew old, she frequently reminded us that she would rather be pushed down the stairs than be unable to enact her own wishes as they occurred to her. It was fortunate for us all that she was able to lead an independent life until she died suddenly from a heart attack.

~

Having a good constitution like hers was a matter of *genetic inheritance.* She didn't understand the process in detail but was certain that for her part, she had contributed the very best to the mix that made us who we were. Admittedly, luck was involved in terms of defects that might lurk in the deep past, and on the *other side,* my father's family. You could not be blamed for bad genes you had inherited, but the person who passed them to you most certainly could.

I grew to understand that beneath all these assertions of health was a visceral fear of sickness and of infection. To me, who grew up in the 1960s and '70s, her terror seemed extreme, neurotic. And I still think so, though I understand now how deeply it was rooted in her experience as a child and then as a young woman during World War II and its aftermath.

Mum's father, doubly sick, suffered and then died from a combination of TB and alcoholism at a time when care for both was primitive and mainly done at home. There would have been heaving and coughing and spitting and bloody handkerchiefs, incontinence, smells. Mum never forgave him for the hard life he had inflicted on my grandmother (a woman never sick herself, no time for it!) or for putting the two women who looked after him at risk: the three of them lived at close quarters in a small row house. In winter, windows were sealed and the large downstairs room closed off to conserve heat. Mum knew without it having to be proved by scientists that poverty and sickness went together. She did her utmost to successfully escape from both, and she succeeded.

But even after that, in the decade following the war, parents affluent and poor alike lived in fear of a child succumbing to polio. Death or ending up with deformed legs or having to lie forever in an iron lung in order to breathe were distinct possibilities.

By the time I was eligible for preschool groups, there was a highly effective polio vaccine. We had to wait until 1970 for rubella. Other, lesser diseases, like measles and chicken pox, were so common as to be almost unavoidable, and in these instances, Mum was a good nurse, dispensing invalid food, treats, and sick-room entertainment. Her expectation was unspoken but clear: thanks to genetic inheritance, our bodies were well equipped to fight back, and we would there-fore avoid the more serious outcomes, just as she and Granny had.

Thus far, my oldest sister's case of rubella, which affected her eyesight, was as bad as things got. Until I became anorexic in my teens, none of us had been seriously ill with anything life-threatening.

As a *mental* illness, anorexia was even more shameful than the physical kind. Was it self-inflicted? Was society to blame? Advertising? Bad genes? (If so, remember, they could only be from my father's side of the family.) Or was it none of those, but pos-sibly some kind of a power struggle between mother and daughter? Absolutely not. The debate over how to assign blame in this case continued for decades after my recovery. Again, I'm grateful, as grateful as I am about not having to tell her about my current unpleasant situation, that Mum lived to her nineties, enabling us to abandon this unresolved argument, and enjoy each other and the later part of our relationship without all the complication.

Anorexia was bad enough, but it did end and I (we) did survive. I suffered neither death nor infertility due to self-starvation, the fates she imagined for me. My New Zealand sister's early arthritis upset Mum deeply, however. She suggested that it had developed because Jan *had used her hands too much.* But this: an adult child of hers with an incurable and progressive neurological disorder? Who might end up gaga, in a wheelchair, both? *Parkinson's?*

I realize only as I write this that Mum becoming convinced of a cause-and-effect relationship between what she saw as the *self-inflicted* mental illness of anorexia and my later developing Parkinson's would have been inevitable. My responsibility for my own suffering would have been clear to her, and that perception would have been extremely difficult for me to bear.

Jan and I laugh now that we do not have to defend ourselves from those fears and accusations, from endless snippets of misunderstood science. But of course, buried deep in each of us and my other, American sister are slivers of the belief that if we are ill, it's our own fault. We made some kind of mistake. What was mine? There could be a link between pesticides and Parkinson's. So was the cause my greedy habit of being unable to resist eating unwashed fruit right from the bag, perhaps laden with pesticides or, alternatively, bacteria?

Reason says no: the value of fruit and vegetable consumption, itself instilled in all of us by our mother, is overall positive, and I think I may well have developed the from-the-bag habit from her. No. Mum's instinct would have been that the fault originated in a character flaw amounting to a moral failing: I had undervalued and squandered the good health she had imparted to her daughters in utero—the greatest imaginable gift. That tendency in me to adopt careless, unhealthy attitudes and behaviours such as staying up too late, being overly "driven" in my various intellectual, artistic pursuits; the way she felt I took things too seriously and did not get proper rest . . . All of that, squandering.

"We are nothing without our health and strength," she'd piously conclude at the end of a discussion of someone else's bodily misfortune, and likewise if one of us had some other grief or loss.

"So, Mum, am I nothing now? Or just less than I used to be?"

"Well, dear, that's just what I mean! You always take things to extremes."

Health and strength went together. Strength was above all about winning, and about never apologizing. A dispute with my father in the car once resulted in her dragging me out of it at the next traffic light and the pair of us setting off on a rainy six-mile walk home. Earning a parking ticket when she had parked illegally to do her shopping, Mum withheld payment, fought it to the highest level, and ended up in custody until my father slunk into the police station to secretly settle her debt. Absurd. Serious too. Mum's refusal to ever admit to being mistaken was fed by and in turn nourished her intense feelings about weakness, physical, mental, or financial. Weakness led to being dominated, to dependency or servitude, erasure, death. She readily acknowledged that the last was unavoidable, but was vigilant and effective in her determination to avoid the rest.

~

Unwanted as it is, most of us will experience a loss of strength and vitality at some point, often long before death. Only some will suffer from the consequences Mum feared, and I am beginning to understand that there are other outcomes, verging on the beneficial, that she did not predict. One of them is that when you are weakened or sick, you may come to understand how much you are loved by those you know and to experience the kindness of family, friends, professionals, volunteers, strangers—even the collective political kindness that created your health care system, should you be lucky enough have one. At the same time, you're almost bound to feel wider empathy, a growth or deepening in your understanding of people whose frailties, slowness, or crabbiness may even have made you impatient before. You learn and become more humane. Everyday interactions seem more fruitful, connective, even revelatory. I'm thinking here of Mary-Ann, or so I think I heard her say when I asked her name, about midway through the half-hour we spent together.

I was walking to the library and noticed her from some distance away: a tiny woman in a red coat, she seemed oddly bent, asymmetrical in many directions and ways, including one foot pointing inward, the other not. I made sure to move into the road, out of her way—the pavement at that point narrows and she was having obvious difficulty walking. I also made sure to look at her and offer a smile, because it's my observation, particularly since I became somewhat more vulnerable physically and very aware that I will become more so, that many people don't see those who are struggling, just as they don't see those begging or unhoused. It's a reflex, largely unconscious: some look obstinately ahead or to the side of people who seem vulnerable or strange; others stop short of that yet manage to avoid contact by not quite focusing on the face. I have been and am still quite capable of doing that, too, but on this occasion did not, so our eyes met.

Immediately she asked, "Can you help me get back to my car?" and as she did so, she stopped walking and held out her right hand.

Yes, I said, of course. I turned to face the way she was going and took her hand. "It's just up there, on the edge of the parking lot," she said. I judged it to be about fifty metres, at most. She took a couple of tiny steps forward, barely able to lift her feet half an inch from the ground. I could feel her arm shaking, or it could have been her whole body. She was wearing well-laced hiking shoes, I noted with relief; they would help her not to fall. "Is that enough support?" I asked. "Or would you be better with one arm under yours, like this?"

"Better," she said. We inched forward. From time to time, I could feel her lose her balance and teeter backwards. But she was very light, and if I held firm, she could self-correct. I thought, of course, of Parkinson's. And then I thought of polio. She could well have been part of the pre-vaccination generation. I asked her if she knew why she was like this. She responded vaguely, saying she hadn't been walking much lately; she'd been doing errands and she must have overdone it today.

"I'm a bit shaky. But," she insisted, "I'll be all right when I get to my car." We were getting closer to that car, but very slowly. Her steps were still tiny, the ground uneven. We kept our eyes on it, looking up only briefly. There were puddles. Since we both wore sturdy shoes we went through rather than around them. I asked her name and told her mine. She mentioned her husband and said he was a good cook. Ahead of us was a road to cross, which naturally had been worrying her. We stood awhile at the curb to recoup and prepare. A white truck coming from the left saw us and slowed to a standstill. Visibility to the right was not great, but we set out across the tarmac and were lucky that nothing came that way.

Three-quarters of the way over Mary-Ann needed to pause. And then the other curb loomed. Some pine cones underfoot. She was breathing hard. We had passed the mailboxes and were less than ten metres from the car.

"I think I'll make it," she said. The closer we got, the more difficult it seemed—she commented on this. I told her to tell me if it seemed impossible. I could probably carry her or get someone else involved if needed. But she was determined. She made it almost to the car, an old but very clean metallic-grey Chevy Impala, handed me the clicker. I pressed, then leaned forward, still supporting her, and opened the door. Held it so she could grab and then lean on it. A series of effortful small shunts, steps, and shifts of grip followed and then she was in and sitting on at least half of the seat. She sat awhile in shocked silence, hands on her knees, then straightened her legs, tested her feet on the pedals. Was she up to driving? If not, if I needed to take that over, it would mean getting her out and round to the other side . . .

But she soon grew calmer and more confident. She wasn't sure if her husband would be home. But even so, home was nearby, and she thought she'd be able to get in, or wait comfortably in the car until he returned. After a few minutes, she wound the window down and reversed carefully out of her spot. She drove a slow test circle around the car park and returned to the exit. I went ahead to check the junction. I was about to remind her to signal left when her indicator light blinked on. A quick wave and off she went, the driver's side window closing as she did so.

Her departure reminded me of that moment when a wild bird trapped and panicking in a room finally finds the opened window—how a part of you soars up and away with it. Sure that she'd get home okay, I set off back in the direction of the library, a mere minute or two away at normal pace.

I noticed how light, indeed happy, I was feeling. It was something to do with having been useful to someone else, and also to do with how close I'd felt to Mary-Ann as we inched our way to her car, and to do with the growing realization that something in me had changed since I lost the vigorous health my mother had endowed me with. Before this, I needed at times to remind or exhort myself to take on the point of view of the sick, weak, disabled, or elderly, to imagine myself into it. I might grow impatient with a slow swimmer in "my" lane at the pool. A wave of selfish irritation might be my first reaction and then I would reason myself out of it. Now, understanding comes more naturally, automatically. I am still fully mobile, but I notice when the wheelchair-accessible toilet is situated at the bottom of a flight of stairs, that the lift to the beach stops by a stretch of rocks, that the cobblestones are dangerous to the point of lethal, and this is of huge value to me.

That there could be any benefits (let alone the positive-thinking crowd's much-touted *blessings*) to be found in being bit by bit ruined by a progressive neurological disease is a notion I have scoffed at in the past and still find hard to entertain. But I do admit that the experience, just like becoming a parent or losing someone you love, offers an opportunity— may even compel a person—to extend and enlarge their sympathies, knowledge, connection to others, and understanding of our shared predicament. The collection of things we call humanity.

In my former healthy incarnation, I'd have helped Mary-Ann, but what I would have understood and intuited of her situation and how to play my part, despite me being a person who in general wanted to do the right thing and be helpful and saw the value of empathy, would have been thinner, more *approximate*. Theoretical, rather than experiential. And Mary-Ann, sensing that, might not have asked that previous version of me to help her, which would have been my loss.

So just as I am glad I did not have to share my bad news with my mother, I now wish I could tell her about Mary-Ann in a way that would cause her to at least pause for a minute or two. Maybe I could draw an analogy with how travel broadens the mind, makes you see and do and feel new things, and opens a window on how many ways there are to live a life. No. I know how much she always loved to come home to her own sheets and brand of tea, how that was such a large part of the point of going away. Instead, perhaps I could tell the story of that half-hour and talk simply about how not being so strong allows you to see and feel and even do new things, that vulnerability might even have some advantages over being *too* strong. How once you accept an unwelcome situation, it may surprise you—

"Well, not me, dear!" she interrupts me to say, pausing a moment to do so, then setting off briskly about the living room to gather up abandoned teacups and plates. And in this half dream of what might have been or might be or almost was, I manage to stop, knowing that she can't or won't see it otherwise, that it doesn't matter which, and it is counterproductive to argue the point. We must leave this topic, these words, even words themselves, however much I love them. I carry the rattling tray of cups and plates into the kitchen and set it down on the counter. Just before she reaches to unhook her apron, I touch her lightly on her shoulder. As she turns, I slip my arms around her, spread my hands wide on her back. I pull her in close, feel her hands reciprocate. She presses her head into my shoulder. I am the taller one now.

17

~

Choosing Delusion

Claudia started the biweekly coffee gathering in the hope of providing her husband with more of a social life. It draws quite a crowd. You don't have to talk in turns or about anything in particular. There's no requirement to be on time or stay for the duration. You can pass the time with one person or flit around. There's free coffee, and you can sample Claudia's baking: today, carrot cake, very good. Coffee, though, is the urn kind. I end up in a small group that's comparing hallucinations, something I've not yet experienced.

"I know that the homeless couple in their sleeping bags are not real. But whenever I glance out of the back window at certain times of day, I see them in the laurel bushes by the car park. They look real, but I know they're not, because my neighbour's dog ignores them, and she would not," Diana says. Did she know it herself right from the first time, or did someone else correct her when she mentioned them? "It's very realistic. I have to think it through," she says. Her face is rather blank, but the sigh she follows this with says a great deal. "I'm getting bored with them," Diana adds.

Stan sometimes hears bits of a radio program after flushing the toilet. It stops when the tank has filled up again and the water is no longer flowing in the pipes. And sometimes he sees women with long hair in flowing garments dancing in the garden. Some are blowing into pipes or flutes. They may be dryads, nymphs, or similar, but he can't hear the music. He, too, knows they're something his brain is producing and do not exist in the actual physical world. To begin with, there was a kind of novelty to it, and they're not frightening or horrific, but he points out that if you want to see what is actually there, it's irritating. He wishes he could find a way to dismiss them and have that shady corner of the garden instead.

If I had an unreal visitor or two, I would probably feel that way, too, but I must admit that from where I am right now, I find all this quite fascinating. Hallucinations, particularly of people and animals, are a well-known result of Parkinson's progression and medications. Stan's and Diana's so far appear only in a particular place, but I discover that some people have a person or animal that may pop up in a variety of places and situations. Parkinson's hallucinations are most often visual, though they can occur in any of the sensory fields—auditory, gustatory, olfactory, even tactile.

What causes them? As ever, no clear answers. It seems likely that either sensory data is arriving in the brain already scrambled and the brain tries its valiant best to make something recognizable out of it, or the faulty brain is persistently misinterpreting sensory data it receives. It's not a surprise to learn that dopamine levels may be in some way involved.

For millennia, some individuals and some cultures have actively sought out such "errors," valuing them as a window into new ways of seeing and being—or even simply as a form of immersive entertainment: the trip. Parkinson's hallucinations need not be especially distressing if the person experiencing them understands what they are. The problem is that they, like the rest of the disease, are liable to *progress*.

While a hallucination is an error in perception, a delusion occurs when someone develops a strong conviction that something is real when it is not and tries to act accordingly. A hallucination can over time establish itself and become a delusion. If the person experiencing it starts to believe in and insist upon its reality, they may be moving toward a form of psychosis.

PWP experiencing hallucinations are therefore advised not to indulge in them but rather dismiss them as soon as they appear. In this respect and in general, it does seem best to have the facts and to base one's choices and actions upon reality. Just as, however tempting an over-optimistic view or however pulled one might be to the negative, expect-the-worst pole, outcomes are likely to be better if imaginary elements and exaggeration are stripped away, allowing us to find a practical way to approach a problem. But there may be some situations where this does not apply. The placebo effect, for example. Neurobiologists studying the complex blend of psychobiological factors that contribute to our ability to imagine ourselves better argue that placebo plays a vital and surprisingly large part in the body's response to proven, effective treatments, to the point that it may account for 50 percent of the benefit patients gain from taking some common antidepressants.

Expectations of benefit from a treatment play a very significant part in the benefit a patient feels from that treatment, particularly as regards reducing pain. The medical rituals surrounding prescription or application of a treatment can increase (or if absent, reduce) the expectation of a positive result. Reduced anxiety based on the simple feeling of being attended to by an expert is also a significant part of placebo.

On the other hand, expecting pain sensitizes the neural system that generates the sensations involved.

While the placebo effect might initially be seen as a kind of trickery, a species of benevolent delusion, its effects are felt, measurable, and positive to the point of life-altering. When we undergo treatment, our own systems interact with and amplify real physiological effects of the remedy. While we may not fully understand it, some of placebo's processes can now be seen at work on the cellular level in the body and brain.

Some might quibble as to whether self-generated effects are a "real" part of a drug's biochemical mechanism; to me, it makes sense to accept that since more than one process occurs when I undergo a treatment, there may be more than one kind of reality involved in bringing about a successful and, yes, *real* outcome.

In the following more personal example of what may be a benevolent delusion, the situation is one I find far more difficult to explain. More than a decade ago, when I still had a sense of smell, a large part of the pleasure and anticipation I used to feel on entering a coffee shop was the complicated aroma: bitter yet almost sweet, not quite burned, almost chocolate, a hint of freshly turned soil, and something, something else . . . I took for granted this tantalizing mixture of the familiar and the exotic until I was confronted with that badly burned pan of rice and realized I no longer had a viable sense of smell.

I'd lost this basic ability so gradually that I'd not noticed what was happening until it was all but completely gone: not just burning food, not just roasting coffee, but vanilla, mushrooms, conifers, cut grass, roses, the smell of rain on dusty streets: an entire sense, a vast and sometimes vital source of information, vanished.

Anosmia, the doctor called it and sent me for a brain scan in case a tumour was to blame. There was talk of chronic rhinitis and a recommendation to wash my nasal passages with saline. My understanding of anosmia as an early symptom of ongoing body-wide neurological chaos came much later, and since I was habituated to my condition by the time I acknowledged it, the feeling of loss was for me less acute than is the sudden-onset anosmia experienced by some Covid-19 patients. I only regret what I am missing when something or someone prompts me to do so. A shop assistant offering me a scented soap or a candle to sniff, my friend moaning with delight as we pass the bakery or jasmine growing in a city garden ... For simplicity's sake, it's often easiest to smile, murmur, agree.

There's irony to be harvested from knowing that according to super-smeller Joy Milne and those who have studied her, we PWP have a very distinctive Parkinson's odour: woody and musky. Could be worse. In any case, I'll never experience it.

There are benefits. Yes, I'm deprived of the sweetness of old-fashioned roses and the fungal tang of rich, damp gardens, and the nutmeg and cookie-jar scent of a baby's scalp; I'm also spared blocked drains, the fumes from the local pulp mill, rotting deer carcasses in the woods, and so on, the downside being that I may not take appropriate action in response to these danger signals unless informed by someone else. Even so, I have larger problems to confront and rarely hanker for the constant stream of pleasure, enticement, and warning that comes to most people via their noses.

I'm curious, though, as to why it is that despite missing an important swath of sensory experience, I do still very much enjoy coffee shops, coffee, and many other scent-related pleasures, including and especially eating.

Neuroscientists are now convinced of something Marcel Proust famously evoked with his dunked madeleine and many of us know from experience: the strong and direct connections between smell, taste, emotion, and memories—bonds far more powerful than that between visual or verbal events and memories. Some scent-connected memories may even be stored not in the hippocampus, where memories are thought to be made, but right in the olfactory bulb itself.

In what sense are memories "real"?

Most research so far has focused on how experiencing a present-day sensory impact in Proustian fashion triggers a deep dive into the past. But in the case of the neurologically impaired, could linkages also work in the reverse direction? From actual situation to aroma?

Another example: it seems to me that when my husband and I embrace, when I press my face into that place where neck turns into shoulder, I still experience, even though it really can't be so, that very particular warm, clean, yet slightly animal scent that has always lived there, and I experience, too, my familiar response to it. Could it be that, since I'm unable to smell, this is a *remembered* scenting experience prompted by the familiar situation, emerging from some as yet intact storage unit in my brain to enrich the current experience? Whatever the explanation, I love that scent.

Coffee, because of its chemistry, turns out to have additional complications, but I wonder, could I likewise have a buried memory of coffee's rather deceptive aroma, a memory just waiting to be triggered by the whirr of the grinder, the hiss and blather of steam frothing milk?

I certainly have fully conscious memories of some coffee-centric moments. One is of my mother bringing me with her to Importer's Coffee on the high street. I was quite young, three or four, perhaps. Child-care arrangements had probably gone awry. Before we even got close came the outrageous smell: a strange, wonderful puzzle you could neither solve nor put aside. Following it, the glamour of the café itself. The waitresses in white aprons, the fancy cups, rows of cakes in glass cases. Then coffee itself, just the tiniest milky sip, begged for—and horrible! How could this be? An embarrassing spurt of tears; Mum and her lady friends laugh and feed me morsels of their various cakes, promise that when I grow up, I'll enjoy the taste of coffee as much as the smell.

True. At fifteen I was, as my mother put it, *addicted*. And *fussy*. As part of the prize for a school writing contest, I ended up on the SS *Uganda* for an "educational" cruise of the Mediterranean. Affronted by the odourless coffee, gritty like diluted mud and served from a huge leaking urn, piano prodigy Angela and I bonded in mutual disgust. Disembarked in Heraklion, we escaped the group and slipped into the alcohol-, cigarette-, and coffee-scented gloom of the first café we encountered. Ordering was more complicated than we anticipated and the men all stared, but soon the coffee arrived, thick as oil, streaming unctuously from tiny pot to tiny cups. We inhaled, sipped, and oh—the sheer, sludgy, impossibly sweet shock of it! Our faces!

A year or two later, I sipped the best cappuccino of my life so far in a café in Soho while my boyfriend haltingly articulated his desire to end our relationship. Torn between hedonism and heartbreak (or was it humiliation?), I chose to detach and focus on the perfection of the coffee I had been served as I heard him out. It's almost fruity richness, just tinged with bitter. The contrasting voluptuous mouth feel of the foam. It carried me through, and I didn't cry until I got home.

I've waited a long time for an explanation of the coffee taste-aroma disjunction that upset me so much as a child. It seems that only the more volatile and aromatic chemical compounds in ground coffee can be detected by the receptor cells in our noses. Careful roasting and grinding adds to the bouquet (but burning spoils it!). Brewing the ground beans releases into the liquid and the surrounding air a class of compounds that only vaporize at higher temperatures.

These compounds are mainly detected inside the mouth by a cluster of scent receptors at the back of the throat and by taste buds evolved to deliver only the absolute basics: salty, sour, sweet, umami, bitter. Caffeine, the effects of which motivate many to keep drinking coffee, is especially bitter—and bitter flavours strongly predominate in these less-volatile compounds. Many drinkers adjust this by adding lactose-rich heated milk, honey, sugar, or artificial sweetener.

We learn to like coffee by connecting or *associating*, as psychologists put it, the bitter and possibly sweetened flavour of the drink with our memories of both the enticing pre-brew aroma and the memory of the enlivening jolt it delivers. As a bonus, once we have made the association between alertness and aroma, studies show that it's possible to attain some of the desired benefits of drinking the brew by merely inhaling the scent of ground beans: another instance of the placebo effect.

In the case of a person who has damage in the part of the brain that normally interprets scents and associates them with other experiences, I find myself wondering, Could it be possible to smell something and react to it *without being conscious of the aroma*? Could the mechanism be working just fine but the *awareness* part be broken? After all, we are all influenced by pheromones without necessarily being aware of them. I have heard from people who've felt horripilation, the hairs on the back of their necks and arms standing on end, when they were in range of a cougar up to that point invisible and otherwise undetected.

In any case, I still go to cafés, smell nothing without really noticing any lack, yet feel a desire for a (glass or ceramic, not paper or plastic!) cup of a beverage that I may only be imagining that I can taste. I make and consume it at home too. Not just any kind: I like it shade grown, organic, ethically produced and traded, interestingly named. I buy beans and grind the correct amount just before I make it. Doing so, I'm not aware of experiencing any aromas. There *is* a taste which varies widely and can be, every ten cups or so, wonderful.

Coffee is said to prepare one's receptors to absorb the medication that keeps me functional some of the time. That would be reason enough for me to consume it, but more salient for me are the pleasures of memory and association.

If I happen to come clean and mention my lost sense, I'm almost guaranteed a query about eating. "Oh, dear. And does it put you off your food? Smell and taste are so strongly linked, aren't they?"

They are, though I bet it's more complicated than it sounds. As for the loss of appetite: in my case, far from it. But I've noticed that a significant proportion of PWP become lean to the point of bony, a natural consequence of medication-induced nausea combined with a diminished sense of smell and therefore taste. Linda from the support group, increasingly skeletal, cites both. She has absolutely no interest in food. It all tastes like cardboard to her. She never cooks but, knowing she needs to eat, buys prepared meals, then forgets to reheat them or loses interest partway. She opens her fridge to show me the contents: a half-eaten plastic bowl of muesli from the local café and several cans of ginger ale.

I've shared several lunches with Stan and his partner, Pat. He's curious, tries most things, but if cake or cashews are available becomes ravenous and eats the latter by the handful.

As the disease progresses, mechanical difficulties with eating—swallowing, choking, control of cutlery, and so on—make it yet more difficult to take in enough nutrition without supplementary feeding. Perhaps our metabolisms change. Our digestions certainly become less efficient. In some cases, weight loss might be at least partly due to the vigorous exercise routines we're encouraged to adopt. Add in tremors, the tense musculature that some experience, and the involuntary movements called dyskinesia: it seems fair to assume that compared to a similar person without the disease, more than normal energy is expended even when doing nothing at all and so more, not less, fuel is required. For some, motivation and capacity just don't match the demand. Doctors, for once, recommend ice cream and chocolate.

I count myself lucky because despite having very little sense of smell, I've experienced no loss of appetite. Indeed, I've never felt as hungry as I have in the past few years, nor have I so consistently enjoyed eating.

Eating is for many emotionally complicated. By my late twenties, I was just an ordinary kind of slim, wiry woman. Teenage anorexia had morphed into normality somewhat tinged with a mild version of what's now called *orthorexia*: an obsession with healthy eating.

Wherever I lived, I grew vegetables, in pots or an allotment if there was no garden. I relied on my father for gardening tips. Colour and visual detail have always been important to me, and I appreciate artistic intent and use of colours in the presentation of food. Nothing is more off-putting than a plate of beiges. But at that time when I was especially keen to consume foods I had decided for one reason or another were healthy, I would overlook ugliness, weird taste, even an outright cardboard-y texture if the nutritional benefits seemed significant. Unleavened spelt bread? Fermented cabbage? Dense green spirulina mixed into a bit of pulpy orange juice? No problem at all; in fact, I came to enjoy the latter in all its murky, concentrated glory, until I suddenly got sick of it. Fortunately, my criteria for "healthy" changed frequently.

Things changed again when I met Richard. He seemed to eat very little during the day and then consume with gusto at night, especially after sex. We ate in restaurants new to me: Japanese, South Indian, Persian. He cooked for us. An incredibly rich onion soup. Grilled racks of lamb; artistic arrangements of sliced avocado, tomato, basil, and fresh buffalo mozzarella on a turquoise plate.

He had low tolerance for ancient grains and chewy bran-like substances and little interest in how good for you a dish might be. He seemed to eat mainly for taste and texture and to be full, for flavours, sensory delight, rather than vitamins. Moroccan dried olives, blini, sea bass in a sauce flavoured with lemongrass, brie, slices of perfectly ripe honeydew melon . . . Also, pizza, baguettes, and other routine things, but the authentic kind with thin chewy sourdough crust, fresh herbs, and so on. My capacity and range of edibles increased dramatically, and I grew more curious about food. I continued growing fruit and vegetables, and so the two approaches deliciously merged.

When tremors and other symptoms began, I became at the same time both incapable of many routine operations involved in home cooking (repeat actions such as chopping vegetables or beating an egg were impossible) and constantly, shockingly hungry. I ate very slowly, prior to the diagnosis and treatment, due to bradykinesia and because my hands became very inefficient and unreliable, so I had to try very hard not to appall whoever might be sitting opposite me. The spoon was by far my favourite utensil. I was secretly glad that Covid meant we never went out to eat.

"It's very weird. I can't really describe it," one friend said when we did eventually share a meal. "It's as if you're from another planet and learning how to do it."

The rest of the family would start to clear up while I finished my meal. I certainly didn't blame them. The bottom line was that until the treatment began to work, I needed an extra meal a day and constant snacks, plus, if possible, dessert (something that had never appealed before) or chocolate. Despite all this consumption, I continued to shrink and found it both uncomfortable and frightening.

Diagnosed and medicated, I gradually regained weight and now do not need a second breakfast. I can chop and whisk and take my turn in the kitchen. I'm still often hungry. When the moment comes, I'm both desperate and hugely appreciative.

So no, I have not lost my interest in food. Logic does suggest that my ability to taste must be taste bud–dependent and rudimentary, yet I don't feel the lack of detail; I frequently have the feeling that what I am eating is delicious.

Granted, I tend to gravitate more to the strongly flavoured ingredients: citrus, mango, chili, turmeric and other spices, garlic, beets, spinach, olives, chocolate, balsamic dressing, oranges, berries . . .

And doubtless my other senses are in overdrive compensating for the absent aromas and more subtle flavours. I've already mentioned enjoyment of colours, shapes, and patterns, whether natural or human-wrought. From the vividness of greens, oranges, yellows, reds to the deep, almost black of tiny lentils to the innuendo of a sliced ripe fig and the pearly shells of oysters. Add to that texture and temperature. A crisp Bosc pear from the fridge. The chewy resistance of a good sourdough, the soft flakiness of perfectly cooked fish, the thick warmth of butternut squash soup . . . It seems to me that a huge amount of pleasurable interest is happening without bothering with smell and taste. I can even relish the sounds in my head as I chew and swallow. And then there is the way food feels and how it changes in the mouth, along with the way eating takes the eater through a little story every time—one I never seem to tire of even though the ending is pretty much always the same: deep bodily gratitude.

Research into the unique and complicated functioning of our sense of smell and its connection with memory and emotion is enjoying a growth spurt. Coupled with the relatively new understanding that our brains are *plastic* (able to adapt and change, to find new ways to achieve a task when destruction or malfunction of part of the brain frustrates the original method), it offers up all sorts of possibilities.

A small number of people with synesthetic colour perception (seeing colours in response to other sensory or verbal information) retain that ability more than a decade after becoming blind or unable to perceive colours.

Could it be that when prompted by the multi-coloured visual glory of food, the chewiness, the crumbling, the warm liquidity, the weight, temperature, the crunch—all that I do still experience with my other senses as I eat—could it be that my brain can bring some stored experiences of smell and taste to enrich my current anosmic experience?

Perhaps at some point ongoing research will illuminate whether and how this occurs. And here at home it would be easy to juice and filter a few vegetables and fruits and come up with a crude DIY test of my ability to distinguish subtle taste distinctions when other sensory information is removed.

But I know that I shan't be doing any such thing. I'm too busy experiencing as much as I can given my progressive condition and the faulty equipment I now possess. Why would I spoil what I still have, a gift horse if ever there was one? Despite a strong preference for realism and being fully convinced of the ultimate usefulness of knowing the facts, in this instance, at this point, I choose delusion, if that's what this is. It surprises me, but I do.

18

~

The Thing I Most
Want to Know

I noticed, among the participants in the online
Parkinson's-specific exercise class, a woman close
to my own age with a thatch of silvery hair and a
direct gaze that made it clear she could be firm as
well as friendly. It was a distinctive and familiar face;
I'd seen her on the news when, as minister of finance,
also deputy premier, she'd deftly fielded questions
about the budget and other matters. Now she was,
like all of us, doing her best to resist disease progression. She was also, I came to realize, very active on
behalf of those with Parkinson's, keen to encourage
and inform.

Apart from some letter-writing, a willingness to
march and protest, and the term I served on our local
school board, my life as a novelist and teacher has
been very different and certainly much quieter than
hers. Carole has been a woman of action constantly
expending effort and working with others to make
much-needed changes while I have engaged with the

intricacies of storytelling and sentence structure. And whereas she is deeply rooted in the community she grew up in, I am part of a family scattered across continents. However, we have both ended up with the same problem, on the same screen in the same class, and now three years later (we're still in the class, run by PWP Victoria), she has agreed to let me join her on one of her daily walks and share thoughts on living with Parkinson's.

I'm excited to meet Carole in person, less so about the conditions: heavy rain worsening over the last half-hour of the drive. Having enjoyed the variety of photographs she has posted of her walks—ocean sunsets and sunrises, wildlife, flowers, but also rain, lowering storm clouds, hail, snow, roiling waves, and her own gale-scoured face and wild, wet hair—I know that we will be walking no matter what.

Carole's house is tucked back from the road, shielded by shrubs and trees. It is painted a subtle clay-pink and looks quite cottage-like from the outside.

She's waiting behind the screen door; her smile beams out despite the gloomy weather, and she welcomes me into a spacious living area.

They moved in two years ago, she says as I fine-tune my rain gear. The house is perfect. It's only a few streets away from the home where she was raised by her mother, stepfather, and grandparents, then later occupied when bringing up her own children. This one is smaller. Granted—she laughs—it's not *small*, but it is a whole storey less than their previous home.

She and her husband, Albert Gerow, an artist and former Chief of the Ts'il Kaz Koh First Nation, can still accommodate the extended family that includes her two adult children and grandchildren, a nephew, twin grandnephews, as well as former foster children with diverse needs, many of whom still love to visit. And, she points out, if needed, the wide staircase will work for a chairlift.

We set off at a medium speed: destination Clover Point via the waterfront trail, with a couple of possible diversions on the way, about four kilometres. Huge chestnut trees about to bloom drip on us as we pass under them. We remind ourselves that rain, given recent droughts and wildfires, is just what we need. Along with, in my case, new waterproof shoes.

~

When Carole was elected as leader of the provincial NDP in 2003, a colleague made her a present of ten sessions with a trainer and urged her to exercise as an antidote to the unhealthy stresses of public life. The habit stuck.

Carole walks daily, first thing. She covers seven kilometres or so and follows up with a shorter excursion later in the day. Since diagnosis, she has added aerobics and boxing classes. Saying this, she laughs, remembering the teachers who knew her as an exercise-avoidant child.

"I go in all weathers. When I was in government, I set out at five forty-five. That was the only way I could fit it in. It's got me through. Now it's seven. Before I've had coffee. Up and out. And of course, living here—" She gestures ahead, where we can see the deeper grey that is the ocean blurring into a somewhat paler grey sky. We both laugh. "It clears my head. It's the only kind of mindfulness I can do."

Ditto with my hikes, I tell her. Could she say more about the head-clearing? Perhaps more used to getting to the point than elaborating, Carole looks for a split second slightly perplexed. "You get going . . . and after ten minutes or so the anxiety drops away into the background. You get back a sense of perspective. You can focus on what's important."

Does she have ideas as she puts one foot in front of the other? Suddenly remember things?

"Yes! Someone I need to contact will pop to mind. I'll rough out the email in my head as I go. At stressful times I often came here, to the breakwater."

Ahead of us the pier reaches out to sea, then makes an elegant curve right toward a small lighthouse. The metal railings, also curved, look delicate in the rain and mist, but beneath them the breakwater is made from granite blocks. Now that it is both safe and accessible, the pier is very well-used. Even on a day like this, it would be hard to turn down the opportunity to walk out over the water. On clear days, you can pause to take in generous views of the ocean, ever-changing sky, harbour, and comings and goings at the cruise ship terminal. Today, we don't linger at the lighthouse but loop back round. The wind now to our backs, we're comparing notes on the neurologist we both see when a well-wrapped older man calls out in passing his best wishes to Carole. She'd be his choice for premier, he says, if only she'd run.

All that is behind her now. The first year of retirement was very difficult. Her work had somehow intermingled with everything else in her life. What was left?

Carole has since childhood possessed a powerful sense of purpose, one that connects her strongly with family and community. She grew up in a large family and thoroughly absorbed the ethic of contribution and hard work. Values, too: her mother and stepfather were activists working to build justice and equity.

Carole did not learn about her Métis father until her twenties and points out that she did not grow up as a member of that community. She is however very clear in her understanding of the need for governments seeking reconciliation to move from dialogue into action.

As a young woman, she naturally took to leadership roles, steadily increasing her scope from local school board trustee to leader of the NDP in 2003; in 2017, when the NDP came into power, she became minister of finance and deputy premier. This was work she had been born and raised to do. She learned how to handle what at times seemed like hostile bombardment during Question Period. Her face and voice became familiar, even to TV avoiders like me. She worked long days, constantly multi-tasking and perpetually in the public eye. And then came the pandemic . . . She knew she was living on adrenalin but coped by sticking with her early morning walks.

We pause to take in a large group of cold-water dippers, many wearing umbrella hats, milling around submerged to neck level in the somewhat restless and clearly sub-ten-degree waters of the rocky bay. Some shivering but jovial swim-suited stragglers wave and beckon us on in. Maybe, one day! Carole says. Cold-water immersion is after all highly recommended for neurological health and renewal.

I'd happily go in here on a sunny day with towels, hot rocks, or even a sauna within reach. But my rain jacket, though recently recoated, is beginning to leak, and my fingers are already numb. I'll give the swim a pass.

In the spring of 2019, during a protracted period of budgetary questioning from the opposition, Carole noticed an irritating tremor in her left hand. Tension or anxiety made it worse, so naturally she blamed overwork.

Come late summer, she and her husband were together at a favourite spot, picking huckleberries. The berries were abundant, ripe but not too soft, easy to reach. She turned slightly to add another handful to the basket—and landed on the ground. Nothing was hurt, but it was strange and unsettling: the ground was flat, the berries required no effort to pick. She wasn't too hot, hadn't fainted. For no discernible reason, she just fell.

Google suggested that this might be a sign of something seriously wrong, but then again, it did seem to be a one-off . . . Until, in the fall of that year, seated in the bleachers at her granddaughter's school concert, she stood to let someone pass, turning a little as she did so, and just as suddenly it happened again.

The diagnosis six months later in early 2020 was devastating, a confirmation of her worst fears. She knew from an earlier experience with cancer how difficult it was to work while dealing with a serious illness and decided immediately not to stand for re-election later that year.

She knew, too, that she would go public about her diagnosis. Because of her public profile, she would be able to draw attention to the disease and the needs of those with it, destigmatize, help people understand. That was quite naturally and without question what she would do, and of course she wanted more time with her family and other loved ones while she was relatively well.

That decision was taken four years ago. Carole recently returned from a walking holiday with three women friends in Portugal and the Azores. Earlier, she took her granddaughter for a week in Paris. Other trips are in the works, and Carole is very much enjoying family—particularly the grandchildren—but finds herself surprisingly busy with work-like activities related to Parkinson's and other causes.

The values, skill set, and desire to improve the way we live together that brought her into politics guide her still in this new life, though with some important modifications. Following the advice of a neurologist, she limits the number of board invitations she accepts, only making a new commitment if she is prepared to resign from an existing one. She declines to chair or lead a committee and selects only a few from the steady stream of speaking invitations. Even so, preparing for these and the other commitments seems, like everything, to take more out of her than previously.

"Your retirement still sounds like a lot of work!" I tell her as, leaving the beach behind, we set off up this walk's only incline.

"You go at a good clip!" she comments. It's the kind of thing we're doomed to notice about each other and total strangers too. The leaning posture, the slight drag to a foot, the one hand that rarely emerges from its pocket: there goes one of us.

She is experiencing new symptoms.

"Anxiety, definitely. Digestive issues. Loss of executive function. I take more time now to organize things. I just can't stand how long it takes me to get out of the house. It makes me mad at myself . . . It's different for each one of us, I know, but there are unwelcome new situations down the line. But you find a way to adapt, and it's better to be proactive and make changes by choice, rather than be forced into them. The first year of retirement was hard. But

I'm glad I scaled everything down. I'm still making a contribution, doing what's possible rather than struggling or regretting the losses, or thinking too much about the grim future. I know it will be a process of constant adjustment . . . But I can keep on contributing," she says. And here it is—behind us the bank of camas flowers, drenched but still a lovely blue, ahead Clover Point—the moment to ask the thing I most want to know.

"Can you," I ask, "imagine doing nothing? Or—how little can you imagine doing? Can you imagine your life without some version of that feeling of purpose? Without doing some kind of purposeful *work* or activity? It's something I'm aware might lie ahead of us."

"I find it best not to think too much about the future—though of course, you need to look ahead somewhat in order to make practical changes and choices," Carole says, as we set off, unable or unwilling in the driving rain to look for the Trial Islands Lighthouse, on the return loop, the quickest, straightest way we can go.

I do take her point. Perhaps the reason I'm so interested in this question is that I had a taste of radically diminished purpose, or usefulness, at the beginning of my illness. I experienced an unusual number of symptoms in a short period of time, and for months on end, there seemed so very little I could do, at least in terms of my sense of what I used to be *for*. How much can our sense of purpose shrink and still be a reason to persist? How much of our sense of who we are depends on work, on being in some way productive? Was I going to have to learn to just *be* with people, in whatever condition I was in? I did not know how to simply *exist*, without purpose or justification. Indeed, it frightened me. My thoughts still return to these questions.

I remember asking Stan from the local support group a similar question. It was only the second time I'd visited, early spring. Lush growth. Hellebores, crocuses, hyacinths, and the shoots of other early plants thrust through thickly mulched beds to either side of the path to the front door—even a potted rosemary bush in flower, in March! How so? Stan shrugged, grinned, informed me that the garden is entirely down to Pat, his partner of forty-five years.

We sat outside in pale sunlight on the wooden deck to the west of the house, rugs on our laps, the rough grass ahead of us dotted with emerging daffodils. Beyond, an open view of meadow, forest, valley, and sky. Stan undertook to make coffee. Pat and I talked plants, trees, new neighbours.

Stan returned carrying one trembling cup at a time and, at the end of it, sat down with care, then leaned back and closed his eyes. He was all right, he said, just very tired.

Fatigue, as some doctors call it, might sound like a genteel and minor symptom, but Stan's and Pat's observation is that it can be one of the most significant and devastating features of Parkinson's. The first of Stan's many naps comes right after he has finished getting dressed in the morning.

"He can fall asleep in a gap in conversation. He once dropped off at the wheel in the few seconds it took a traffic light to change. Terrifying! We agreed that he won't drive. He's surrendered his licence."

Stan raised his cup, met her eyes steadily over the rim.

"And the falling. It's very dangerous. I won't leave him alone overnight. When I need to be away, one of our sons comes to stay."

The shadows crept closer. We moved our chairs a couple of metres to the left, changed the topic.

I'm curious, very curious, I said, as to what Stan thinks and feels about the need for purpose. The legal work he used to do must have provided it in spades. Has he now found a new way to feel he's contributing, making some kind of difference, or is that something that he has found he can or must live without?

At some point, even those who retire voluntarily confront a changed sense of purpose and altered identity. Some take the hedonistic "bucket list" route or develop hobbies or help with their grandchildren. Others throw themselves into advocacy, activism, fundraising for research, setting up support groups and so on. I think of our friend Linda, who began the local support group. Of physiotherapist Jill Carson who closed her practice when Parkinson's affected her ability to work. After a year or so of confusion and denial, she brought her experience to bear and founded Parkinson's Wellness Project, the organization that offers at an affordable (or no) cost the Parkinson's-specific exercise programs that Carole and I both attend. Others move into fundraising, offer bookkeeping services, and so on. There are many who, like Carole, make use of skills developed in their former lives, scaled down to a doable level, and throw their remaining energy into community, into making life better.

But eventually that may become impossible. Can we get used to not having a driving purpose—to not being, in any obvious way, *useful*? Could that even be a good thing? Or at least an interesting thing? Could existing without busyness and justification for being alive turn out to be a release and a relief after decades of focused, productive activity? Could learning to be without all that be an unexpected benefit of this situation? Or am I clutching at straws here, trying to turn something that may be personal to me into a bigger thing than it is?

There was a long pause after I'd offered this tangle of a question to Stan. I realized his eyes were closed. I had bored him to sleep! But no.

"There are certainly people who argue that purpose is something we *should* live without," he replied, eyes still closed, and he muttered some names that I later found I'd forgotten to record. Unlike Pat, he added, shifting in his chair, opening his eyes, he has no spiritual affiliation. Being part of a community is the best remedy he has found (and, I recall him saying the previous time we talked, it was something he felt he had lost in the move to this smaller place). As for contribution, he signs up for research studies, most recently one on diet. "It's important. But," he added dryly in his hoarse almost-whisper, "doesn't quite compare."

The shadows lengthened further, but we stayed put, fell silent, stared for long moments at the trees and sky and grass. Pat reached for the binoculars in the side pocket of her chair and focused on a moving speck that had alighted on one of the mature firs their new neighbour was angling to cut down for the sake of his view. Three deer appeared to the left, in the sunny part of the meadow. They looked up at us and briefly froze, before lowering their heads to eat.

"Did you know the mother uses her tail to signal to her fawns—to warn them of danger? I love watching them," Stan said, and I remembered then how when my father's mobility declined, he increasingly depended on watching the world go by—people-watching especially. His observations were acute, and he took a deep pleasure in sharing them. He had become part of life's audience.

For a few moments there at Pat and Stan's place in the spring, I felt a vast, amorphous pleasure in the ability to perceive, in my privileged location in a part of the world where there's still so much life, so much to observe and in that quiet way, yes, be a part of.

I was going to try to say some of this but by then Stan *was* asleep, his head dropped toward his chest.

Months later, to my surprise he returned to the question, presenting me with a framed print he had bought years ago in Santa Fe, a mixture of drawn figures and hand-printed text. *It may be*, says the writing at the bottom-right corner, *the real reason we are here: to love each other and eat each other's cooking and say it was good.* I have it on the wall in my office.

~

On the return leg of our walk, my recently resurfaced breathable waterproof jacket now a wet shroud, Carole and I look more to the landward side, at glassy new apartments, a few holdout character homes, apartments, the occasional quirky hotel or society hall, and talk about how we both chose early on to connect with others in varying stages of the disease. Not everyone with a new diagnosis wants to do this, far from it, but, she says, "It's very valuable to me. I see people living great lives despite terrible losses. It's really surprised me."

I, too, am grateful to have been shown how individuals and couples come to terms with ongoing unwelcome change—to be blunt, how people suffer and adapt. How relationships alter and new ones are formed, how some find happiness in the most unlikely-seeming ways and places.

And here again, as our walk comes to its end, it is fascinating and perhaps reassuring to realize that this brave politician and I, so different in many ways, have come to many similar conclusions and at this point both feel, each in our own way, that we are still doing something meaningful.

What's interesting is that when a scaled-down reality is accepted, doing what is now possible doesn't feel like a lesser thing at all. And so, logic suggests that if what is possible should lessen effectively to nothing, that, too, might seem just fine, or perhaps very interesting. Or even be a kind of happiness?

I'm even more curious now than when I began to think about this. I'm no longer so afraid. I'm hopeful, almost to the point of being certain, that I'll meet my answer in due course. But first, Carole suggests, some tea and a dry-off while we wait for Richard to arrive? And so it is that I leave wearing a pair of her favourite Danish hiking socks.

19

~

Progress in Progression

I bought an e-bike early in the summer of 2023. I was wary because it seemed like an admission of defeat, but at the same time I was keen, verging on desperate, to try something new. Recently retired from the university, I dedicated my last shrunken, quarter-time salary payment to the purchase of the most budget-friendly option, a Milano Plus in matte white, powered by a lithium battery, capacity: 48 volts, 16 amp-hours.

"But what do those numbers mean?" I asked Max, the bike shop's lanky manager who, summer and winter, spends all day in his cycling clothes, a kind of perpetual advertisement.

"Well," he began, "voltage is a bit like the pressure in a pipe—"

"Sorry," I said. "What I meant was how far will a full charge take me?"

"Good question!" Answer, rather vague: anything from fifty to one hundred and fifty kilometres, depending on many factors including the terrain (very hilly), the way I rode—especially how much electrical assistance I required—and the weight of the bike plus me (27 kilograms + 52 kilograms = 79 kilograms). How these factors might collectively merge into an average number of kilometres per full charge was, well—he smiled and shrugged—"impossible to say."

I decided *not* to ask Max about lithium, now so very much in demand for making batteries but also useful in many other ways—including as a powerful antipsychotic drug that is currently, at microdose level, the subject of small-scale trials for the treatment for Parkinson's. Because of its market value, this soft, silvery, wonder-metal has become a source of human misery and ecological destruction wherever it is extracted from the earth.

"You'll develop a feel for it," Max concluded confidently. "Same as with coordinating the gears with the assistance. On the island, so long as you're fully charged, you'll be fine for anything you'd want to do."

I paid up and rode home at alarming speed.

An alternative starting point for this story might be fifteen months prior before we had moved, in February 2022—I often struggle to pinpoint the beginning of something, whether a story or a shift or change of direction in my own life. I am reliable as to the order and linkage of events, but my experience of time has always been subjective and elastic. Having Parkinson's has not helped.

In any case, at that point I'd been taking carbidopa/levodopa for over two years. We took a short holiday, our first since before the pandemic. Like everyone else, we felt we'd been through a lot, so feelings of relief and excitement as well as our expectations for the trip ran high. We set off early one morning for the ferry to Vancouver Island and then drove on increasingly empty and poorly maintained roads past glimpses of old growth, lakes, and clear-cuts to Tofino.

At the end of the drive: cold, clear air, an immensity of light, a vast glittering ocean, and a wind-scoured beach as near empty as we remembered it. The cabin was warm. We cracked the windows open to better hear the breathing of the waves.

But the next morning when we were walking on the beach, I noticed that my left arm had forgotten what to do. It was supposed to swing, reaching its furthest forward point just as my right heel hit the ground, doing so at the same time as the right arm reached the highest point of its backwards swing and my left foot left the ground. This sounds complicated, but most people do it with no awareness of what they are accomplishing. My right arm and left leg, however, were doing just fine and probably felt rather smug. The other half of my team had lost the plot.

All this had happened before, way back in 2019 before diagnosis and before the medication sorted things out. It was one of my first symptoms and was associated with walking at a slower and more companionable pace. I remembered Richard telling me, when I asked how noticeable it was, "Well. It looks like something's *wrong.*" Were the gains I'd made since starting the carbidopa/levodopa treatment beginning to desert me? Was this the beginning of the end of the so-called honeymoon period? Two years? Too soon.

I could still *somewhat* fake it: I could remind my left arm to swing in a kind of replica of what it was supposed to be, but I could not produce a natural, loose, unconscious walk. My attempt on the beach that morning was stiff and military, and probably comical as well as unsustainable. I relapsed the moment I stopped attending to it.

At the same time as faking arm swings, I was struggling to be part of a conversation I could barely hear and trying to reassure myself.

My legs still carry me along perfectly well. Nothing hurts. An uncooperative arm is a small thing. Yes, but— *Sitting in the car all day always messes me up. It always takes awhile to recover. Why fixate and magnify?* Because it's my body! I live in it!

The delinquent arm reminded me of that word I so dislike: *progression,* which sounds like a blend of *progress* and *procession* and so rather celebratory, but means, from the point of view of the disease's unwilling host, that things are getting *worse* for you while the illness thrives and does what is in its nature to do. My disobedient arm was a messenger, an advance guard, preparing the ground for all the unwelcome changes impossible to fix or conceal that lay ahead.

Richard reached for my hand to hold, my *left* hand, and I pulled it away.

"What's up?" he asked, and we stopped walking.

"Are you noticing my stupid arm?"

"Well, yes. A bit wonky today. Is it bothering you?"

"A bit. A lot. Yes." We stared at each other. Was I crying, or were my eyes watering anyway? He reached out his arms and I hid in them. I did not have to explain that knowing he, too, had noticed my gait made it a bigger and more important sign; had he been unaware, I might have been able to minimize it for myself. But even so, yes, I did and do prefer an honest answer.

We walked on in the miraculous February sunshine. I thrust both hands in my pockets, a good disguise, but it did not stop me from covertly examining the other beach-walkers we passed. I envied them all, despite whatever problems they faced unbeknownst to me. I envied them what I supposed was their lack of self-consciousness and for the thoughtless way their legs kicked forward, how their leading feet struck the ground heel first, how the foot rolled, gently pitching them forward until the other foot detached, heel first, lifted, kicked forward, and took over. Most of all, of course, I envied their arms' effortless coordination with these so well-behaved opposite legs and with each other, back and forth—such easy, generous swinging! That they could take it for granted.

Even as I did all this envying, I knew how unhelpful and self-indulgent yet also self-defeating it was and what a waste it was to be technically present on the beach we'd travelled all of a day to reach, but actually caged inside my untrustworthy body and my fears for the future. I was furious, too, mostly with myself. What to do? Scream?

Just before dusk, I slipped out alone onto the beach. The tide, about halfway out, had left a broad expanse of firm sand, marked only with the footsteps of birds. I ran as hard as I could to the rocks at the end. No arm problem at all! I ran halfway back, boiling in my windproof jacket. Unzipped, I jogged: likewise problem free. Even walking was good!

For an hour or so, it turned out. Better than nothing. Perhaps things were not as bad as they had seemed.

The next day, a tanned, windswept young man in a plaid shirt and artistically threadbare jeans showed us a tiny hut, the beach sauna, already hot inside. He pointed out the water dipper, then took us round the back to the woodpile and the stove, demonstrated how to keep a steady temperature. There was an outside sitting area, a cold outside shower. Last of all, he waved at the ocean: a long way out but in his opinion plunging in it was not to be missed. He wished us well before disappearing down a trail into the woods.

The two-hour session was a surprise joint-birthday gift from our daughter, Becki. Stripped down to our bathing suits, we reclined on the towels spread over the hot cedar planks. We tossed water as instructed and gradually became invisible to each other. Periodically one of us slipped out to the back of the hut to stoke the iron stove, then, shocked by the cool air, hurried back and stretched out to sweat again until a moment more seemed impossible, at which point we burst gasping and salmon-fleshed into the chilly outside, each outlined by a full-body halo of steam. There was no question, though, that we would honour Becki's gift and at least *try* the ocean plunge.

The tide was low and the slope of the beach gentle to the point of non-existent, which left no choice but to splash-run on water-coated sand toward the distant ocean expanse, eventually meet the chilly silver wavelets, then keep going, caressed by a freezing wind, until the cold gripped at mid-thigh. There we launched ourselves in, shrieking. In an instant, the water devoured what remained of our body heat. Every capillary, appalled, squeezed tight. Keep moving! One minute, two, and then blessed numbness . . . We fled back toward the sauna, our wind-whipped skin now blue-tinted blotched lobster, purple, yellow as if bruised by the brief immersion; when towelled, our skin ignited with a strange, cold blaze. Euphoric, we gladly repeated our ordeal twice more: steam, sweat, dash, plunge, freeze, burn, dash.

Remember, I told myself later in my notebook, how it felt when my entire attention was absorbed by sensations—then and later, too, when we walked back along the beach, napped, made love, ate the fine food we had cooked at home, and finally slept like rocks. Remember that; leave the rest behind.

~

At home, news of the war in Ukraine, of children killed. Communities pounded to rubble. Catastrophe. Appeals. All you could do was donate. It didn't stop, and in March snow fell, melted, refroze into an icy plaque that hid treacherously beneath fresh falls. And April lived up to its reputation: dead land, dull roots, mere glimpses of a veiled sun. Brave snowdrops, clenched daffodils, blossom buds tight on cherry trees. No point in preparing to sow or plant.

Meteorologists used the phrase *Arctic outflow*. The climate crisis intensified, *progressed*, as did the war. Talk of supply chains, the global food supply unravelling.

I hadn't been able to use the driveway, icebound, then slush-buried, to practise my sprints and jumps. Higher trails were impassable. So yes, there were perfectly plausible explanations as to why my routine had gone to the dogs since the previous September when I'd hit my best-ever time for the forty-yard dash: 8:03 seconds. I knew this because my achievements were meticulously recorded day after day in a series of tiny field notebooks.

Not only exercises, but everything I did from typing to hiking had become more difficult. Much of me began to hurt, a new development. However much I stretched, the large muscles of my legs seemed perpetually taut, the tendons hawser-like.

Even by mid-May when everything had dried out, I did not improve. But—but—but—there were the stresses of our imminent move, then the aftermath of it, all the changes . . . It was surely possible that these things were at least partly to blame?

"Stress may be a factor, but I don't think it's the entire explanation," my neurologist said. "Unfortunately, this is just the way it goes."

"It's your choice," he said when I declined the increased dose he was suggesting. "But take the prescription. Just so you have it there if you change your mind." He said *if*, not *when*, though the meaning was clear. He recommended a specific physiotherapist, a woman my daughter's age. (This made me like her.) I should start from where I was, she said, not from where I used to be. Change things up. Find new ways to elevate my heart rate. Cycling?

She was right. The ancient exercise bike parked in the new backyard had been good for interval training, but I did miss the landscape unfurling, constant change, freewheeling down a hill I'd ground my way up. I missed the bumpy roads I'd once enjoyed, before such outings ended in sweaty defeat. But there it was: an e-bike, not a *real* bike. Assisted cycling. That degenerative, losing-ground feeling. Yet what else was I going to do? I had a real bike and wasn't using it.

So I bought the bike from the Lycra-clad man in the cycle shop, and I rode it all summer and into fall.

One October morning so gorgeous that I could

not stay inside as planned, I climbed onto the e-bike and made for the nearest trailhead—a steep but brief uphill ride. The display showed one bar of charge remaining. Probably enough.

I cycled along the shady, tree-lined road that leads out of town, up through a zone of gentle hills, and rises more steeply as the mountain proper begins. On the first stretch, I drew nothing from the battery. When I turned onto the suddenly steeper lower slopes of mountain, it looked as if I still had pretty much all of that last available bar of power on the display. A few minutes later, breathing heavily but not gasping, and using significantly more assistance, there was still more than half of that bar. Plenty!

The winding route offered constantly changing views, sometimes of the ocean, sometimes of building sites or lots for sale, new houses sprouting solar panels, the first signs of food-producing gardens, ambitious orchards on near-bare rock. I enjoyed taking in the details of the landscape until, just before the left turn into the parking area, electrical assistance deserted me.

My pampered legs took too long to adjust. The bike teetered to a standstill. I had to push it to the trailhead. More amused than anything, I realized as I locked the bike to an alder tree that in my haste to get out into the sunshine I'd forgotten to bring the daypack where I keep not just my phone and water bottle but also the medication due at noon—which was fast approaching.

It would have been sensible to return. Also depressing. Instead, I set off through dappled alders into forest lush with mosses and ferns. The hike has a gentle start. As the gradient increased, I could not ignore the telltale tight resistance-band feeling in my legs, the beginning of the thing called *wearing off*. I was running out of dopamine. However much I ordered my legs not to shorten their stride and however hard they tried, they could not obey—not without a pill.

The truth was that at the best of times, this sensation—this sudden exhaustion, the unwilling legs, the loathed tendency to trudge and generally economize on effort—was becoming increasingly familiar at around half past eleven, as much as half an hour before the next dose was due. On that October day, I felt all that together with a vacuous, panicky feeling and an inner shakiness that threatened something worse still might break through if I did not get that foolishly forgotten medication down my throat and into my brain.

Halfway up the next incline, I had to pause again. Why was I doing this to myself? Did I need something like this to make me finally concede to reality, admit that I was running out of juice? That this was happening to me and I needed to take some kind of action.

Until then, some part of me had unconsciously hoped, or even believed, that since I did the right things, put in the effort, I would be one of those few

Parkinson's sufferers who manage to yield only the smallest amount of ground to their uninvited guest.

But virtue is not always rewarded. Marooned on the slope that day, I knew that I would not be one of the lucky few. I was not going to be a PWP who would stabilize and stay on the same dose of medication for ten or twenty years, for whom progression is "like watching paint dry." I would not make use of a supposedly dual passport, would be forced instead to inhabit this other country, the kingdom of the sick, for the duration.

I resumed the uphill trudge, surprised to feel a fragment better mentally if not physically for levelling with the facts. Were there any other positives to be gleaned? I told myself that while my efforts might not have worked miracles, they had thus far helped everyone to feel better about the situation, including me. Maybe a period of denial was sometimes necessary, even helpful? And I would probably have been in worse shape, had I not tried. Though admittedly this achievement was difficult to appreciate as I forced myself joylessly up the uneven, dusty trail— or even when weak, dizzy, and hot, I stood on the summit, looking out across the water to Vancouver Island, its spine of mountains basking in the sun.

Resting there awhile, I thought of how when we hug after a hike, my artist friend still tells me, admiring, encouraging, or both, what a *warrior* I am. I don't feel that way at all. How much does she see? And others? I didn't know or want to ask.

I took a gentler trail slowly down to where the e-bike waited, powerless, a dead weight. What a pair! Just as I inexorably lost my dopamine-producing neurons, so with each recharge, a few of the battery's lithium ions fail to return to the cathode and so over time the amount of charge that can be accepted diminishes, and battery capacity decreases.

Heigh-ho. Giddy up! One failing machine, riding another.

I confide in one of my Parkinson's acquaintances, also a writer, Len. He's had it for over a decade, lives hours away. We've never met in person, and we're not close. Perhaps that helped. We usually email, but for this I call.

"Have you told your man about this?" he asks. He means my neurologist.

"Not specifically. He'll say what he said last time: increase the dose or the frequency. Or take another damn thing. I don't want to!"

"Isn't it a bit late to object to pills?"

"Admitting defeat," I tell him, "makes it all much more real." Though in a battle known to be of the losing variety, what exactly *is* defeat? Len doesn't bother to argue that point. He could, but it would be beneath him.

"I see no good reason," he pronounces hoarsely, "to deny yourself relief if it is available. Get real. You are going to have to take what you can get. For heaven's sake, go to the pharmacy."

~

And now, months later, having benefitted from the physiotherapy, purchased the e-bike, and caved and cashed in my neurologist's latest prescription, I'm somewhat bewildered by the fuss I've made. Groping my way toward an understanding that accepting I am fighting a losing battle, yet doing so with some kind of grace and style, could be a form of liberation, a victory of sorts, or at the very least more fun and more interesting than trying to ignore what is happening. I'm back where I started, with Viktor Frankl and Anatole Broyard.

The neurology office at the top of the building has huge windows and basks in light. We're surrounded by a baby-blue sky just a few shades lighter than the stripes on my neurologist's shirt. Insulated windows eliminate traffic and other noise from below. He is seated in the super-adjustable chair behind his enormous desk; I'm in one of the two armchairs, also rather large, parked in front of it.

"How is it going?"

"I did use the prescription, thank you, and it has helped." A nod, a quick note. "I do realize that it's best to accept the facts. As you said, it's the nature of the beast for things to get worse.

"Unfortunately, yes."

"I thought I had, but part of me was really hoping to be a special case." I notice, shocked, that it feels verging on good to say this. What's going on? Am I hoping for a gold star? "Well, there are bad days," I tell him, "but still, plenty to do, enjoy, and be interested in. I'm meeting some extraordinary people ... I think I've almost finished my book. A draft, I mean. A bit later, I may have some science questions to ask you." I could be imagining the all-too-understandable flicker of panic on my neurologist's face, but in any case, I stop there. I refrain from lyrical gushing about the many blessings in my life, loving my husband, children, friends, strangers, moonlight, frog song in the spring, and from trying to explain the excitement generated by even an occasional glimpsed possibility of new ways of seeing and being. I don't want to seem like an advertisement for a disease.

"Looking ahead," he tells me, "there are still options to explore." *Options. Explore.* It sounds quite attractive. "Other drugs, perhaps. Different delivery systems. Pump delivery of levodopa straight into your upper intestine, for example." A bag of gel worn round the waist all day. A nozzle to sterilize every night. Not so exciting ...

But there's more: "You could possibly be a candidate for evaluation for deep brain stimulation, but only when your symptoms are considerably worse. Of course, not everyone is suitable, and there are serious risks." One of which, I know, is "verbal imprecision": slurred and dysfunctional speech. So, a risky surgery involving electrodes implanted in the brain via holes drilled in the skull, the undeniable effectiveness of which has not yet been explained? Well, yes, actually, I could be interested in that. Or rather, I know I might become so, when I get to that point. That's the way it seems to work.

"Good to know," I say.

"Yes. What else are we monitoring . . ."

"Well, my degenerating left side balance is definitely worse, especially when other things are worse too." This is ongoing, nothing much to be done. "The twitchy foot—"

"Dystonia. We've already a plan for that. Any falling?"

"No."

"Very good. Keep it that way." A pause. There must be something else I need to say or know, but I'm too exhausted to remember it.

"Questions?"

"No, not right now. Thank you." I reach for my bag, stand ready to leave.

"You are doing very well," he says as our eyes briefly meet. It surprises me how touched I am by this seemingly simple and now familiar acknowledgment. I don't care to quiz him as to exactly what he means by it: physically or psychologically? Both? Something else? I do know that this is a different *very well* to the previous *very well*s. It means very well *for the new situation*. At this point, I'll take it with many thanks and no quibbles. I hope to do my best at getting worse.

~

20

Endings Are Also Difficult

Now in my fifth year as an involuntary citizen of the kingdom of the sick, I share the feeling, common among older people, of time not merely passing but accelerating. We feel on our backs the hot breath of Apollo's four horses as they drag the sun god daily across the sky; where on earth, we ask each other, does the time go?

Those with serious or progressive disease are additionally aware that the period during which they will continue to be to some extent *living well* shrinks at a yet faster rate—considerably faster than it does for others of their age.

When all this began and I didn't know what was happening to me, what to do, or how long it would continue, time seemed to stretch around me, an edgeless, interminable miasma. Days and weeks brought no new information, direction, development. I was preoccupied with what was happening in my body. Other important events in our lives and further afield faded into the background, making it ever more difficult to sense the passing of time. I realize in retrospect that this loss contributed a great deal to my feelings of loneliness, of exile. I was not the same as other people, could not do or think as they did. My mind was full of things I could not or chose not to communicate, that I did not want to inflict on others, but also feared articulating and sharing because doing so would make my feelings and the unwelcome information I was accumulating seem more real. I did not fully grasp at the time how very lonely I felt. The image of sudden expulsion, a border crossing into another country, of separation from the well, expressed this in a powerful, visceral way.

That first year, capable of very little, I found that recording my experience in note form was a small thing I could do, and it had no impact on others. Being an observer slightly separated me from my predicament and oh-so-tentatively reconnected me to my former self. It suggested a future, one unlike the present—a time when the notes I wrote might be of *use*.

It began to seem to me that what I was going through, particular as it was and continues to be, offers a perspective on an experience most people in affluent societies will at some point confront, whether via sudden illness, a frightening diagnosis, long-term disability, or the creeping erosion of physical and mental powers that comes with aging—that dreaded disintegration or diminution, or both, of what we used to think of as ourselves and the way that it changes us, our relationships, our understanding of life, and how we want to live it. I hoped and still hope that my experience, if—given diminished resources—I could find a way to portray it, might be useful to others.

The physical act of writing continued to be difficult and painful. I had the beginnings of carpal tunnel, along with limited mobility, painful hands, and ongoing shoulder pain that worsened with mouse use, most of which was to correct typos. Later I was to learn that a frozen shoulder is a frequent precursor to Parkinson's in women.

I'd lost dexterity. I could not press a pen or pencil hard enough to make a good clear mark. Ghostwriting took on a new meaning. My touch typing, never more than adequate, became glacial, and even then my hands sabotaged my intentions. Wayward fingers inverted the order of letters, struck neighbouring keys; thumbs went into overdrive inserting random spaces in the middle of and after words.

I obeyed the physio and purchased ergonomic equipment for my office. In the hope of re-establishing the failing connection between brain and fingers, I embarked on a touch-typing program and, with daily practice, saw very gradual improvement. Later, I tried a much-recommended dictation software, but the combination of my new, flatter voice and my rather more British than Canadian accent seemed to confuse the software. Teaching it to hear me properly would have been a torturous process that took longer that I felt I had. I resigned myself to turning out a few painful but finished sentences at a time. Simple depictions of what was occurring.

Why write at all, especially given the difficulty? Would it not be of more value to be out and about, soaking up experiences, doing every wonderful and outrageous thing still open to me, rather than typing slowly in a quiet room? Good question—I'll say only that I don't seem to work that way.

So, looking beyond possibly self-deceiving altruism, why write this thing? Stubbornness. Blind persistence. A desire to thumb my nose at the disease by creating something of value from the destruction it inflicted. A way to hang on to my former life. While I can imagine not writing—I have thought it through in some detail and believe it might be workable—I'm in no hurry to test this hypothesis.

In my second year of treatment, my dopamine level having increased and stabilized, I grew more physically functional, and both the thoughts and feelings I had and the sentences I needed in order to express them became more complex. I felt more pleasure in writing. The scope and aims of what I wrote broadened beyond capturing a life-altering experience in words. It became a kind of enquiry, a way to dig into the reality of Sontag's "other place" and my reactions to it. Using a form new to me, creative non-fiction, helped me to explore and focus, and to consider the many questions I had, such as what my new citizenship might require of me. I asked myself, *How do I do this?*

Writing was and is a large part of the answer.

~

About two years ago, as we settled into our seats at the support group, I asked my neighbour how she and her husband were doing. I will always remember how she drew breath, paused, puckered her mouth as if tasting something sour, and replied carefully, evenly.

"We recently calculated that eighty-five percent of our interaction with each other is to do with Parkinson's." She was perfectly still, yet the whole of her seemed to vibrate. Outrage, I sensed, and grief. She held my gaze while I floundered as to what to say, then summed up for herself: "Horrible."

Carers, mainly spouses, now move to their own room for the second half of the support group session, with a facilitator for their meeting. Sometimes we hear a loud burst of women's laughter. Sometimes they all emerge in tears.

Richard and I have got to know this couple over the past three years and are very fond of them both. Even though he prefers not to join the group at this point, Richard has a kind of honorary membership: he comes to set up the technology when we have visiting speakers. Given what a small place we live in, he has met many of those who attend.

~

A month later, we're invited to lunch at their home. Rich colours, wide-open views. From the beginning, the mood feels lighter, even though, as they recount it, the situation is the same, or worse. Day-to-day life is increasingly difficult and unpredictable. Frustrated, confused, depressed, he falls often, though so far with only minor consequences. She is unable to lift him if he cannot get back up by himself. Terrified he will seriously injure himself, she can't leave him alone for more than an hour or, at most, two. She is desperate for a break. It can't go on like this. Together they have resolved to explore and test out the available options.

"A matter of choosing the least bad of a poor selection!" he points out. They feel best about the idea of hiring a professional carer to come in for several hours, perhaps three days a week. If that works, she'll be able to go to yoga or coffee with a friend, knowing someone competent is there and that he has someone to talk to. And she'll have something to talk about when she returns; they'll chip away at that 85 percent. The experiment starts next week. When we look to him for corroboration, he nods, yawns, already exhausted.

And, she adds, they have things to look forward to this summer, especially their son's wedding. The bride's mother helped her choose a sari. Would I like to see?

Remembering this conversation later, I realize how important that moment was. What I have written so far, because of its focus, may have failed to convey a simple but important aspect of the situation: for anyone with a progressive disease, progression and losses are impossible to ignore, but even so, the experience of disease is rarely absolutely *all* of life, even when it *almost* is. At times it fades for a period, brief or long, and may be for a while almost forgotten.

Large parts of our lives are merely touched upon in these chapters. Richard has curated art shows, taken singing lessons, organized a speaker series, sung to a rapt audience, become part of a band. I have taught classes, retired, written this. We left our former home, adjusted to our new one. We've taken control of, or rather *liberated*, our new garden. In the early summers, we've swum in silky lakes, and later when it is truly hot, in the frigid ocean, afterwards spreading out on hot sandstone to warm through and dry, hearing the slap of waves and the voices of children playing on the shore. From our own backyard, we've seen meteor showers and eclipses, even, once, the aurora borealis. We've been horrified by wildfires and windstorms, smoky skies that obscured the sun.

My New Zealand sister, artist and birdwatcher, visited us last year: a wonderful surprise. Prior to that, we travelled with our daughter to Spain and from there to Richard's niece's wedding in London.

Recovery days were needed, but I was able to spend time with friends who have known me for decades. All this happened alongside meeting new people of all sorts, reading hundreds of books, and watching some excellent television drama.

I've deliberately written very little about our children because they prefer it that way. My sickness has not affected our ability to support them through various crises, changes, and choices. We've celebrated their achievements and enjoyed their growing agency and their company, continually wonderstruck: such kind and intelligent people! As to what lies ahead of them on this heating planet ruled by slackers and maniacs? The unfolding of their lives will likely be a source of terror as well as wonder. In the past five years, the world has become far less physically and politically safe—increasingly authoritarian and frightening.

After the lunch with our friends, Richard and I help to clear up. It's been such relief to see them looking lighter, happier. He's napping. The three of us are sorting leftovers into containers when a sudden clatter interrupts us. Nap over, he hurtles toward us, bent forward, legs at frantic double time, hands reaching toward the countertop.

"Stop!" she yells as he crashes, grabs, holds tight. "You know how that scares me!" His chest heaves. Is that a grimace or a grin I see on his face? A kind of manic glee?

"Calculated . . . risk!" he says. "Easiest way."

She wipes her eyes with the back of her hand.

Months later, we catch up again at the support group. None of the three carers they tried has worked out. Now, she says, they are trying the day program at a local long-term care centre. In the circle, we shuffle our chairs closer, lean forward, strain to hear.

"Misgivings? Yes!" he says. "Spending all that time with people who . . ." A long pause. "Even worse mentally than I . . . . Frankly, demented." He looks around at our faces.

"This is just a trial," she says. "To see what it's like."

"Turns out some are very interesting to talk with . . . or observe. Music . . . art . . . games . . ." He shrugs. "Bingo!" At this, his eyebrows shoot up and the volume and clarity of his voice double. "I just don't understand! A passive game entirely without strategy! *No* thinking needed—no effort of any kind! Just sit there. You can have someone check your numbers. I may have a few suggestions . . ."

"It is just a trial," she reiterates.

"The staff are kind," he adds. "Very kind."

Sometimes, on one of the program days, she and I hike, talking as we go about mutual friends, gardens, books, writing. In a blink, months evaporate.

We're at their place again. Cake plates and crumbs on the table. She looks carefully from him to us and back as she explains to us that he has decided to put his name on the waiting list for a place in the local residential care facility.

The wait will be about eighteen months. Which gives them time to unravel the financial impact. She might not be able to keep the house. It seems from the way each reassures the other as they tell us about the decision that they are holding on to the core of the relationship they have built. There's respect, regret, tenderness.

The facility has a good atmosphere. It's run by the same kind people as the day program.

"But the rooms are very small," she says. "I don't think I—"

"It's only for sleeping," he says.

This, then, is the least unpleasant option in the circumstances? Hard, I feel, to imagine anything worse. How on earth to make the best of it? We are in shock; they seem to have moved beyond it. As much as the decision itself, it is the way these two, a couple for forty years, seem to have made it together that makes both Richard and me tearful on the drive home. In the note I send afterwards, I struggle to express the depths of our admiration for them.

Richard and I have been together for almost thirty years. Naturally, our relationship has changed over that time, adjusted, fine-tuned itself. It's based on messy reality, and we have a deep, practical, flaws-and-all kind of love for each other. Hugely important is that I know I can talk frankly with him. I trust him completely. I think I always have done, ever since the creative writing class I taught when he slid into the last chair, exactly on time.

When I most recently told him so, it was, I must admit, a precursor to asking if he felt the same about me. Absolutely, he said, always.

Now, I tell him again what he already knows: a care home, even one run by kind people, is a line that from here—intermittently functional, wineglass in hand—I cannot imagine crossing. It's not only that I resist what I imagine to be, kindly run or not, a drab, overregulated, overheated, lonely, boring existence with awful food and long gaps between yearned-for visitors. It's also that the diminished version of me that might have to move there is not how I want to be remembered. And I'd rather our children and theoretical grandchildren were able to inherit whatever this solution would cost. What would they rather have though?

"In any case, Jim won't let us!" Richard reminds me. We laugh, remembering the vehemence of our son's proclamation, made after a stint as an aide in residential care. Such a thing would never happen, he declared, even if it meant dropping whatever he was doing to come and take care of us. We shan't hold him to it.

On the other hand, some years back our daughter made it equally clear that she did not intend to wipe parental butts. We would not wish the task on either of our grown-up children. But I know that what often happens is that as you draw closer to the thing you thought would be intolerable, you start to see its advantages. What was once unthinkable, impossible, becomes acceptable, even desirable. The new form of us betrays our former self. Or you get beyond thinking at all, and then it's too late for medical assistance in dying, should you want it, or have wanted it when last you were coherent, should it be available where you live.

Choices, choices. First-world problem. May never happen . . . Stay aware, we beg each other. Keep talking.

As for our friends, "I'm afraid those nice things you wrote about us aren't always true," he tells me weeks later, clearly distressed.

"Stupid arguments," she explains when I ask, waving her hand as if that could drive them away.

A bad patch.

Of which there are plenty. Caring 24/7 for your partner, my friend writes, *has its rewards, I suppose, but would not have been my choice. How Parkinson's changes one's life . . . can't be predicted. In my experience, it can bring out the best and the worst of a relationship within the blinking of an eye.*

It's difficult to talk about rewards, compensations, or unexpected benefits of suffering, given that any such outcomes, however treasured, have come without negotiation or consent at outrageous cost. Yet those I know—PWP, partners, families and close friends—when confronted with the damage and unattractive choices Parkinson's presents them with, do for at least *some* of the time deepen their understanding of and commitment to each other. Many endure and find ways through things they didn't think they had the capacity for. Likewise, we find ourselves drawn or pushed to discuss topics and consider actions previously avoided. We learn about ourselves and each other. In my experience, this has been unexpected and of great value.

I have become more intimate with some of my friends; I trust and love my husband differently, more deeply. I treasure my New Zealand sister. Such ongoing mutual support and easygoing, affectionate honesty. Such pleasure.

Difficult circumstances push some to reach beyond their normal circle—to form new friendships and connections. Carers who offer each other practical help and emotional support in crisis come to care for and love each other. But how does this weigh against their losses? Is such a weighing possible? I think not, and I'm also certainly not recommending this unwelcome predicament as "character forming," much less as a "gift" or a "blessing." What I observe is simply that as well as being painful, destructive, and very sad, the situations we are forced to deal with can strengthen and burnish our relationships.

I remember a warm summer evening spent at a free concert in the park. Balkan Schmalkan were playing to a willing crowd of young, old, and everyone between, including several people from the support group. A dozen or more performers filled the stage—percussion, cymbals, woodwinds, all kinds of brass—pumping out a crazy fusion of Roma music, klezmer, jazz, and pop, laced with passionate if incomprehensible-to-me lyrics in Serbian, Romani, and Italian. The music twisted and shimmered, played with being martial, lapsed into chaos, turned lascivious, became a tipsy wedding march. Soon there would be no choice but dance. As the first people abandoned their chairs or rugs and drifted to the grassy space between stage and audience, Richard and I glimpsed a couple we'd once known in a professional context years ago, then met again in the support group. I knew he had Parkinson's but not how bad it was. He had become unnaturally still, increasingly locked in, absent-seeming—in complete contrast to his vivacious wife whose features expressed every shift and lift in mood, who could not hear music without moving to it, who enjoys life so very much.

That evening, she led him in a strange but wonderful dance in the space in front of the stage, her green dress flaring and swirling as she amplified the small movements he could make and combined them with her own.

I don't, of course, know whether they were enjoying each other and felt in that dance as free from their ongoing difficulties as we, watching, wished them to be.

I began this account with the metaphorical acquisition of an unwanted passport to that other place, the kingdom of the sick, as proposed and elaborated upon by Susan Sontag, Virginia Woolf, Rebecca Solnit, and others, including me. I found the metaphor very useful, particularly early on. But all metaphors have their limits. I'm aware now that there are many aspects of the situation which the idea of exile to another place fails to express, or even contradicts or conceals.

For the most part, sick and well live among each other in the same homes, streets, and towns. We are married to each other and otherwise in many ways related. Beyond the intimate bonds of family and friends, we share the same streets, parks, doctors, and hospitals, water and air, governments, media. The idea that we reside in separate kingdoms does not reflect this complicated reality. The initial shock of serious illness may make the two states *seem* poles apart, but as my experience continued, that feeling dissipated. Should some of the well not understand our situation, or avoid doing so because of fear, if they don't seem to be aware of our experiences and needs, then it falls to us to forge connections and diminish ignorance. Begin conversations. Consider how to handle uncomfortable reactions. How to gently remind the hale and healthy that frailty does at some point come to most of us. Ask what might we all, both sick and well, do to improve life for those who are vulnerable. Commit to the situation, to each other and to the strangers on the beach, to projects that aim to diminish fear and ignorance, dissolve artificial borders, and make things better than they are.

I would shred that passport but seem to have already mislaid it.

I've always been a painstaking writer. At the peak of my relearned typing skills, I was still very slow. Now on the downside of that peak, I've recruited a team to read, eliminate typos, and enable me to keep up some sort of pace.

My hopes for these dispatches continue to grow. They may be inflated or unrealistic—readers, if any, will judge—but I'll take the risk of admitting at this point that I am well past writing this only for myself. I do want my account of these five years to be of use to others; to be, as certain books have been for me, a source of both inspiration and consolation. It is my hope to connect with both the sick and the (so far) well, to stimulate further connections between them and beyond, to spark further curiosity and increase mutual understanding.

I write also to celebrate some of the many people I've met, talked, laughed, wept with, and learned from, and to spotlight the ingenuity, persistence, generosity, humour, courage, dignity, and bloody-mindedness that I see in fellow PWP and those close to them. Doing so has necessarily involved conveying something of the nature of what afflicts us. I hope I've made it clear, though, that the disease is not and never will be the star of this show.

Author's Note

~

Nothing in this book is intended as medical advice, and any errors are my own.

In This Faulty Machine is a work of creative non-fiction. Faithful to my experience of events, it is written from memory and notes, both of which are fallible if perfect accuracy is at issue: we do all unconsciously shape both our actual experience and the memories or stories we make and remake from it. I have also consciously made some changes for the sake of narrative flow (for example, combining several conversations on the same topic into one). As for the people who appear or share their own stories in the narrative (as a former novelist I find it hard not to write *characters*), those who have an extended presence read and graciously approved of the relevant pages. While some people are referred to by their real names, others have preferred or been given a pseudonym and/or I have changed them in some ways so as to make them unidentifiable.

Acknowledgments

In This Faulty Machine would not exist were it not for the openness and generosity of those whose observations and stories form an essential part of the book. I am equally grateful to family, friends, professionals, and colleagues who supported me by reading individual pieces or even the whole typo-strewn manuscript (in some cases several times) and sharing their responses, questions, and encouragement. I will mention in particular my sister Jan Linklater and my husband, Richard Steel.

Writers Caroline Adderson, Vicky Grut, John Metcalf, Shaena Lambert, Betsy Warland, and Brett Josef Grubisic, along with my Island friends and community, and—from distant undergraduate days—Ricky Lowes: all these and more formed what I eventually began to call "the team." Some read the entire manuscript or parts of it in several iterations; some painstakingly corrected typos only to have me create more of them in the revised drafts that followed.

John Pearce of Westwood Creative patiently waited several years to see a full-length manuscript, keeping to himself any doubts he may have had about my ability to complete the project and meanwhile providing succinct and useful feedback. He then directed the book to the desk of Lara Hinchberger. Working with Lara has been a revelation. I am profoundly grateful for her calm support and dedication to the text. It has been a great pleasure to have someone so very well-read understand and appreciate the book, then offer acute observations that enabled me to deliver the final draft.

My thanks go also to Crissy Boylan for her sensitive ear and eagle eye, to Vaani Sai Nagallapati, and to all the kind and skillful team at Penguin Canada. Publishing is hard and complicated work and without them the book would be a lesser and a messier thing, or perhaps not a book at all.

I offer heartfelt thanks to Bailey Martin and all the staff, volunteers, and fellow participants at the Parkinson Wellness Projects in Victoria, who have kept me moving with exercise classes and at the same time provided a source of up-to-date information and a place of understanding, community, and connection. PWP has had a huge impact on my quality of life.

Last but far from least, I am grateful to the British Columbia Arts Council for vital financial assistance that enabled me to complete and revise this book.

Sources and Suggestions
for Further Reading

CHAPTER 1: PASSPORT

Susan Sontag, *Illness as Metaphor*

Virginia Woolf, *On Being Ill*

Haruki Murakami, *What I Talk About When I Talk About Running*

Oliver Sacks, *Awakenings*

Oliver Sacks, "Oliver Sacks: A Neurologist At The 'Intersection Of Fact And Fable'" (Highlights of NPR Interviews with Oliver Sacks from 1985 and 2012: published online in 2015)

Hanif Kureishi, *Shattered*

CHAPTER 3: THE MAN IN THE RED-LIGHT HAT

Jo Marchant, *Cured: A Journey into the Science of Mind Over Body*

CHAPTER 4: AMPLITUDE

Wei Li et al., "Suicide in Parkinson's Disease," in *Movement Disorders Clinical Practice*, Volume 5, Issue 2

Angela L. Ridgel et al., "Forced, not voluntary, exercise improves motor function in Parkinson's disease patients," *Neurorehabilitation and Neural Repair*, Volume 23, Issue 6

CHAPTER 5: TROUBLE WITH WORDS

Raynor Winn, *The Salt Path*

Elena Semino et al., "A Metaphor Menu for people living with Cancer" (Lancaster University; the menu can be found at https://wp.lancs.ac.uk/melc/the-metaphor -menu/)

Shaena Lambert, "Oh, My Darling," in *Oh, My Darling: Stories*

Harold Macy, "The Beast Within," pp. 190–200 of *All the Bears Sing*

Francois Gravel, *Colonel Parkinson in Charge*

Peter Dunlap-Shohl, *My Degeneration*

Hilary Mantel, "Meeting the Devil," in the *London Review of Books*, Vol. 32, No. 21. The essay is also collected in her book *Mantel Pieces*

Eula Biss, "The Pain Scale," *Seneca Review*, Spring 2005, Vol. XXXV, No. 1

Rebecca Solnit, *The Faraway Nearby*

Anatole Broyard, *Intoxicated by My Illness: And Other Writings on Life and Death*

Eve Joseph, *In the Slender Margin: The Intimate Strangeness of Death and Dying*

Sarah Manguso, *The Two Kinds of Decay*

Jean-Dominique Bauby, *The Diving-Bell and the Butterfly*

CHAPTER 8: OH, DOPAMINE!

Daniel Z. Lieberman and Michael E. Long, *The Molecule of More: How a Single Chemical in Your Brain Drives Love, Sex, and Creativity—and Will Determine the Fate of the Human Race*

Alison Abbott, "Levodopa: The Story so Far," in *Nature* 466

"Researchers discover a potential cause of Parkinson's disease" (summary at www.helsinki.fi/en/news/brain /researchers-discover-potential-cause-parkinsons -disease). Original report: Vy A. Huynh et al., "Desulfovibrio bacteria enhance alpha-synuclein aggregation in a Caenorhabditis elegans model of Parkinson's disease," *Frontiers in Cellular and Infection Microbiology*, Volume 13

A. Lopez et al., "Mechanisms of the effects of exogenous levodopa on the dopamine-denervated striatum," *Neuroscience* 2001

Asociación RUVID. "Dopamine regulates the motivation to act, study shows," at ScienceDaily, 2013

Kent C. Berridge and Terry E. Robinson, "What is the role of dopamine in reward: hedonic impact, reward learning, or incentive salience?" *Brain Research Reviews*, 1998

Colin G. DeYoung, "The neuromodulator of exploration: A unifying theory of the role of dopamine in personality," *Frontiers in Human Neuroscience*, 2013

Giulia Enders, *Gut: The Inside Story of Our Body's Most Underrated Organ*

CHAPTER 10: BE HERE NOW

Matthew D. Sacchet and Judson A. Brewer, "Advanced Meditation Alters Consciousness and Our Basic Sense of Self," *Scientific American*, June 2024

CHAPTER 11: CHRONIC

Jesse Barron, "Completely Without Dignity: An Interview with Karl Ove Knausgaard," *The Paris Review*, 2013
Philip Roth, *Letting Go*
Ottessa Mosfegh, *Eileen*

CHAPTER 12: HOW DO I DO THIS?

Leesa S. Davis and Matthew J. Sharp "Preliminary Notes Towards a Comparison of Stoicism and Buddhism as Lived Philosophies." https://www.academia.edu/13037452/Notes_towards_a_comparison_of_Buddhism_and_Stoicism_as_Lived_Philosophies
Viktor Frankl, *Man's Search for Meaning: An Introduction to Logotherapy*
Thomas Szasz, *The Myth of Mental Illness: Foundations of a Theory of Personal Conduct.*

CHAPTER 15: A CURIOUS TALE

James Parkinson, *An Essay on the Shaking Palsy*
Andrew Lang, *The Blue Fairy Book.* Lang's source for Bluebeard was: Charles Perrault's "La Barbe bleüe, *"Histoires ou contes du temps passé, avec des moralités: Contes de ma mère l'Oye.* For exploration of the Bluebeard story and how it has been interpreted,

see "Bluebeard and the Bloody chamber" on
Terri Windling's blog at www.terriwindling.com
Further sources, on curiosity: Ian Leslie, *Curious: The
Desire to Know and Why Your Future Depends On
It* and Marret K. Noordewier and Eric van Dijk,
"Curiosity and time: from not knowing to almost
knowing," *Cognition and Emotion*, Volume 31, Issue 3

CHAPTER 17: CHOOSING DELUSION

Benjamin D. Young, "Smelling phenomenal," *Frontiers
in Psychology*, Volume 5

Anne-Marie Mouly and Regina Sullivan, "Memory and
Plasticity in the Olfactory System: From Infancy to
Adulthood," in Anna Menini, ed., *The Neurobiology
of Olfaction*

Megan S. Steven and Colin Blakemore, "Visual synaesthesia
in the blind," *Perception*, Volume 33, issue 7

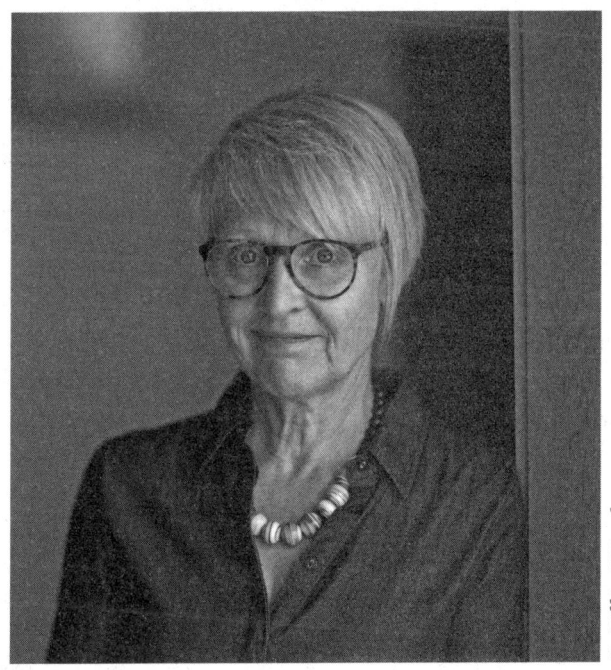

KATHY PAGE is the author of eleven acclaimed works of fiction. Her books have been twice nominated for the Scotiabank Giller Prize, once for the Orange Prize, and shortlisted for the Governer General's Award and the ReLit Award. Her most recent novel, *Dear Evelyn,* won the Roger's Writers' Trust Fiction Prize, the City of Victoria Butler Prize, and was a Best Book of the year for *The Globe and Mail, Kirkus, Quill & Quire, Toronto Star,* and *Winnipeg Free Press.* Born in the UK, Kathy has lived on Salt Spring Island, BC, since 2001.

As for the ups + downs, no clear rationale.
All I can say is:
① Stress or anxiety makes it worse
② Exercise for an hour in the morning improves
whatever the baseline is. Trying for better
sometimes works (As with "wrote bigger."

"Good" days are few + far between. Today the co-
from or when walking was better than it has been
weeks. I took no propanolol yesterday + am plan
do a few days without. and see what happen
beginning to wonder if it was actually making
worse, + does a) affect arousal staring b) make for
extremities.

                                    SAT 6th Feb
                                      ½ day 2

                        sleep interrupted
                        on waking — good

                        Tremor — low key but +

                        Walk — unchanged

                    *   Co-ordn — medium

                        H-writing - unchanged

                        Arm stiffness - low key but

                        Slowness - unchanged
                        Bowels - I trustful I were
                    *   Driving first thing feels easie

                    *   mid aft best.

                        I do of exercise. again

list of gifts. Good. pen friends thank you
friend J. comments to write so I
gifts, for holidays me in
hamster (intended meeting
more subtle!)